A Diet of Reason

A Diet of Reason

Sense and Nonsense in the Healthy Eating Debate

Edited by Digby Anderson

Published by the Social Affairs Unit

Book production by Esmonde Publishing Limited

British Library Cataloguing in Publication Data

A Diet of reason: sense and nonsense in the healthy eating debate.
1. Nutrition 2. Health
I. Anderson, Digby C. II. Social Affairs Unit
613.2 RA784

ISBN 0-907631-26-6

ISBN 0-907631-22-3 Pbk

Typesetting by TJB Photosetting Ltd., South Witham, Lincolnshire
Printed and bound in Great Britain by SRP Ltd., Exeter

Contents

The Authors:

Dr. Digby Anderson is currently Director of the Social Affairs Unit. Previously he was Research Fellow in Health Education at the University of Nottingham where he studied the effects of dietetic interviews. His books include *Health Education in Practice*, *The Ignorance of Social Intervention* and *Evaluating Curriculum Proposals*. He has also published numerous papers in journals including *The Sociology of Health and Illness*, *Health Education Journal*, *The Philosophy of the Social Sciences*, *Journal of Curriculum Studies* and *Sociology*. He is a regular columnist in *The Times* and writes a food column in *The Spectator*.

Dr. Barbara Pickard is an Honorary Research Fellow in the Department of Animal Physiology and Nutrition at Leeds University. She has written extensively for both the popular and scientific press about nutrition and pregnancy. Recently the increasing trend to condemn meat and dairy products as being damaging to health has led her to review the literature on the subject.

Professor Donald J. McNamara received a Ph.D. in biochemistry from Purdue University, Lafayette, Indiana and worked at the Rockerfeller University from 1974 to 1985 on clinical studies of the regulation of whole body cholesterol metabolism. He is at present Professor in the Department of Nutrition and Food Science at the University of Arizona in Tuscon. He is a member of the American Society of Biological Chemists, the Council on Arteriosclerosis of the American Heart Association and the American Society for Clinical Nutrition

Professor J.D. Swales was appointed to the Foundation Chair of Medicine in the new Medical School at Leicester in 1974 and has been Head of the Department of Medicine there since then. He is a Fellow of the Royal College of Physicians and the High Blood Pressure Research Council of the American Heart Association and an Honorary Fellow of the Australian High Blood Pressure Council. He is a past Editor of the *Journal of Clinical Science* and immediate past-President of the British Hypertension Society, Secretary of the Association of Clinical Professors of Medicine, Pro-Censor of the Royal College of Physicians, an Executive Council member of the National Kidney Research Fund and a member of the Clinical Research Panel of the Wellcome Foundation. He is Editor of the *Journal of Hypertension* (the official journal of the International Society of Hypertension. He has published widely on sodium metabolism and clinical hypertension and has lectured throughout the world.

Professor Ian Macdonald is Head of the Department of Physiology at Guy's Hospital. He is a past President of the Nutrition Society and is currently Chairman of the British Nutrition Foundation. He was Chairman of the joint WHO/FAO Expert Committee on Dietary Carbohydrates and is at present a member of the MAF Food Advisory Committee.

Professor Vincent Marks is Professor of Clinical Biochemistry at the University of Surrey and Head of the Department of Clinical Biochemistry and Nutrition at St. Luke's Hospital, Guildford. He is a Fellow of the Royal College of Physicians of London, the Royal College of Physicians of Edinburgh and the Royal College of Pathologists. He is best known for his work on the investigation and treatment of disease of carbohydrate and fat metabolism but is also known for his work on alcohol, drug addiction and his early advocacy of therapeutic drug monitoring and the bringing of clinical laboratory testing nearer to the patient. He is the founder Chairman and Director of Guildhay Antisera Ltd., a University-based corporation specialising in antiserum production.

Marshall Midda graduated from the Royal Dental Hospital of London and, after a period in private practice and as a specialist in the RAF Dental Branch, became Consultant Dental Surgeon and Director of the School of Dental Hygiene at Bristol Dental Hospital. He is a past Chairman of the British Dental Health Foundation and a member of the Board of Directors of the International Academy of Peridentology. He has published and lectured extensively throughout the world to professional audiences on the subject of preventive dentistry.

Dr. Reg Passmore is retired from the Readership in Physiology at Edinburgh University. He has been a Consultant for the FAO and WHO in South America and Thailand and a member of their Expert Committees on Nutrition. He was for many years a member of the Food Standards Committee of the Ministry of Agriculture and of the COMA Committee of the DHSS. He is co-author of *Human Nutrition and Dietetics* which has been the standard British textbook for over 25 years. The eighth edition (written with M.A. Eastwood) was published in 1986.

Professor Anthony R. Leeds graduated in Medicine from the Middlesex Hospital, London in 1971. He worked at the MRC Gastroenterology Unit on nutrition-related problems before moving to Queen Elizabeth College (now King's College, London) in 1977 where he teaches nutrition and supervises research on dietary fibre and obesity, while still continuing clinical practice.

Dr. James Le Fanu is a doctor and medical writer. Educated at Cambridge and the London Hospital, he spent eight years in hospital medicine before being appointed Medical Editor of the Medical News Group in 1982. In 1985 he returned to medical practice but continues to write on a freelance basis for the *New Scientist*, *New Statesman*, *The Economist* and *Daily Telegraph*. He has written extensively on the pharmaceutical industry, cancer therapy, embryo research and diet and disease. He has also acted as Medical Consultant to the independent television company, Meditel. He has taken a special interest in heart disease both in practice and at a theoretical level, contributing to the debate on its causation in the pages of the *British Medical Journal* and *Lancet*.

Charles Plouviez worked in the Festival of Britain before joining a medium-sized advertising agency as a copy writer, retiring 32 years later as Chairman. For five years he was Chairman of the Advertising Association's Public Affairs Group. He is now a freelance writer and consultant to various voluntary organisations.

Catherine Montgomery Blight and Simon Scanlan are both on the staff of the School of Agriculture, Edinburgh. Mrs. Blight is a solicitor and economist with a special interest in regulation and agricultural policy. Mr. Scanlan is an agricultural economist specialising in livestock marketing and agricultural policy.

The opinions expressed in the chapters of A Diet of Reason *are those of their individual authors and not those of the Social Affairs Unit. But the Unit is pleased to be able to publish them as a contribution to and extension of an important public debate.*

Glossary

Since *A Diet of Reason* is intended for the intelligent layman, technical terms have been kept to a minimum and when they do occur, most are intelligible by context. However these brief explanations may help.

Aetiological	causative
Atherosclerosis	thickening and rigidity of the arteries in the body associated with infiltration of the walls of the arteries with deposits of cholesterol
Blood cholesterol	the concentration of cholesterol in the blood
Carcinogenic	a substance capable of inducing cancer
Colon	the part of the bowel that connects the small intestine to the rectum
Demineralisation	loss of the minerals calcium and phosphate from the bone, leading to a thinning of the bone
Diverticular disease	disease of the colon in which pouches of the bowel protrude
FAO	Food and Agricultural Organisation
Fibre	the non-digestible component of cells of plant origin
Haemorrhoids	'piles', inflamed condition of the veins around the anus
Hydrogenated	fats chemically treated by the addition of hydrogen molecules
Hypercholesteraemia	a high level of cholesterol
Hyperlipidaemic	a high level of fats in the blood
Hypoglycaemia	a low level of glucose in the blood

Intervention Trials	scientific studies in which the benefit of a proposed treatment is tested by giving it to an 'intervention' group, and comparing the results with a 'control' group
Intraluminal colonic pressure	the pressure within the colon that pushes forward the contents of the bowel
Intussusception	a type of obstruction of the bowel in which one section of the bowel slides into the part immediately beneath it
JACNE	Joint Advisory Committee on Nutrition Education
Metabolic ward studies	scientific studies of the effect of changes of diet on small numbers of patients, performed on a hospital ward
Mucosa	the membrane that lines many of the hollow organs of the body and secretes mucus
NACNE	National Advisory Council on Nutrition Education
P/S ratio	The ratio of the amount of saturated and unsaturated fat in the diet
Plasma cholesterol	the concentration of cholesterol in the plasma
Saturated fats	fats from animal or dairy sources
Unsaturated fats	fats from vegetable or fish sources
Volvulus	obstruction of the bowel produced by a twisting of a loop of the bowel around itself
WHO	World Health Organisation

1 Healthy Eating: the Evidence

Digby Anderson

1 No justification for simplistic messages about 'good' and 'bad' foods fired indiscriminately at the whole population

The British housewife, her husband and their children are currently bombarded with messages telling them what to eat to become, or stay healthy. The messages on radio, television, posters, labels and in books and pamphlets come from farmers, food manufacturers and processors, qualified and unqualified nutritionists, government-funded bodies, journalists, cookery writers, medical bodies and academics. Many of their authors have obvious axes to grind, for example the food manufacturers. But there are less obvious motivations and less obvious motivations are often more dangerous. There are academic scientists with ambitions to political advisory posts or in search of research money following publicity, mundane journalists for whom food scares about 'our increasingly sick society' provide an easy source of revelatory stories, other politically-motivated journalists keen to discredit 'capitalist' food producers, government-funded bodies forever seeking to increase their perceived influence and consequent grant. And those who seem to be on the side of 'progress' in the fashionable forms of bran and yoghurt are as likely to be motivated by financial reward as those who defend plum pudding.

It all amounts to a healthy competition in information in which the competitors busily scrutinise and criticise each other's claims and the consumer learns to discount the exaggeration typical of such a competition. The trump card in the game is science. All the players, not least the man and woman in the street wanting to feed themselves and their families in a healthy way are constantly looking for the piece of scientific research which will 'prove' that by eating more or less of this or that, by following this or that simple diet we will all avoid disease and live, if not forever, at least much longer. In such conditions discriminating readers of dietary advice would do well to treat anyone claiming to have such a card, such a piece of research with a certain wariness – with more than a pinch of salt.

In particular, there is one group in the healthy food debate which claims to have conclusive evidence about healthy eating and is so convinced of its own opinions that it sees no need for further debate. It is time, it says, for its opinions to be imposed on the population by specific government policies. The continuation of the disagreement and competing claims of the public debate are unnecessary, even harmful because scientists, it says, now *agree* about what constitutes a healthy diet. These 'scientists' are said to have conclusive evidence, on the interpretation of which they agree, that the British people all eat too much meat, fat, sugar, and salt and not enough fibre; that many of them are dangerously fat and that their eating habits cause major killing illnesses such as heart disease. The group urges a radical change in national diet so that we can all reduce the risk of such diseases and live longer, healthier lives. This is to be achieved by the Government funding propaganda on 'healthy' eating and banning the production and advertising of foods the group decrees to be unhealthy.

In their different ways, the authors of *A Diet of Reason*, reject this position. The evidence relating diet to health is not conclusive. Indeed much of what is presented to the public even in supposedly official reports such as that of the National Advisory Council on Nutrition Education (NACNE) or by quasi-official bodies such as the Health Education Council, is not strictly scientific. There is no single clear, simple message about fat, salt, sugar and fibre or even about body weight agreed and packaged by scientists and ready for popular dissemination. There is no guarantee that if we change our diet to avoid allegedly unhealthy foods that all, even many of us will enjoy better health let alone live longer. Indeed some such changes might even make some people less healthy. Interference by the Government in the agricultural market has so far led to the production of more not less 'unhealthy' foods and it is better to leave the choice of what to eat to individuals. Banning advertisements for foods decreed 'unhealthy' would not help wiser eating.

In short, the public is being deceived by those who push a simplistic health message identifying good and bad foods for all in the name of science and arguing for Government food controls. The state of scientific knowledge does provide much on which thoughtful consumers might ponder. There is a case for a balanced diet. Some individuals need specialised advice. There is a need for health education. But there is no justification, scientific or otherwise for crude propaganda about supposedly bad and good foods fired aimlessly at the total population at public expense.

2 Dairy products and red meat: denounced by the media and 'experts' but not by the findings of research

Dr Barbara Pickard severely criticises those who go beyond the evidence in trying to link consumption of fats in milk products and meat with heart disease. Giving a wealth of contrary evidence, she argues that organisations such as the Health Education Council should preach the attested virtues of balanced, moderate eating rather than invent categories of 'healthy' and 'unhealthy' foods inconclusively supported by scientific evidence. Different age, income and other population groups need different advice. Ill-informed advice to reduce meat consumption may reinforce malnutrition in certain groups. And advice which is scientifically unsupported and subsequently shown incorrect destroys scientific and medical credibility in matters where there is good evidence.

3 Heart disease: fat consumption not a proven cause

It has been traditional to stress the importance of the quality of food eaten, the balance of foods and moderation. This is being currently replaced in public awareness by a good-food/bad-food attitude in which some foods such as fruit and vegetables are held to prevent disease while others such as fats cause it. Professor Donald McNamara's chapter shows, as do others, that scientific, particularly epidemiological research has failed to provide hard evidence of a direct cause and effect relationship between single components of diet, in this case cholesterol or saturated fat and heart disease. Nutritionists and dietitians cannot say precisely which fats and oils elevate or reduce blood plasma cholesterol levels in individuals.

Heart disease is caused by many factors not all of which are known. And who is at risk? Studies show that a generalised message to the public may encourage the many to change their fat intake needlessly but not result in adequate changes among the few who might benefit. A general renunciation of eggs or red meat is not the answer. We need to identify the few individuals at risk. They might need to do more than give up eggs.

4 Fibre: too much speculation, not enough facts: weak evidence on preventive benefits, possible harmful side-effects

If fat is allocated by the modern food propagandists to the bad-food class, fibre is a star among the 'good-foods'. Yet Professor Ian Macdonald points out, the evidence of its beneficial effects is far from conclusive. The link between high/low consumption of fibre and bowel disease is, at best thin, being often based on comparisons of widely differing societies in which many other, possibly contributing factors also vary.

Certainly fibre intake has been statistically associated with the low incidence of some diseases but it has also been associated with a higher incidence of others (stomach cancer). Two conditions in which fibre is therapeutically useful are diverticulosis and diabetes. But in neither case is it known to be preventive. To advocate that all the population eat more fibre when its preventive effects are not known and there is a possibility of harmful side-effects is not responsible medicine or nutrition.

5 Salt: not the universal villain but given a bad name by misinterpretations of source reports

Professor Swales reaches similar conclusions about salt. It is often thought to be a bad food contributing to high blood pressure but in fact though reduced salt intake may, when combined with some other treatments, lower the blood pressure of patients with very high blood pressure, 'for the remaining patients and the rest of the population it seems to have little effect', nor is it established that too much salt is the cause of the high blood pressure. Why then have others come to different conclusions? The main example of such different conclusions is the report of National Advisory Council on Nutrition Education. Swales shows how this misinterpreted the sources it used and indeed selected these on an inadequate basis. More generally he is concerned with the pressure to pronounce immediate solutions to highly complex problems; solutions which may have harmful effects.

6 Sugar: 'toxicologically safe and nutritionally acceptable', certainly not a cause of juvenile delinquency and hyperactivity

Professor Vincent Marks contrasts the pronouncements made about sugar by health propagandists with the scientific facts. The propagandists try to link sugar consumption especially that of white sugar with diabetes, heart disease, obesity, hypoglycaemia, dental caries and even behavioural disorders such as delinquency and hyperactivity. But except in the case of dental caries the evidence is thin and in the case of the behavioural disorders laughable. 'There is very little evidence that the increased consumption of sugar (sucrose) is really responsible in the population as a whole, for producing any disease apart from caries of the teeth.'

7 Sugar and dental caries: no simple link

Even with caries the link is not simple. Marshall Midda explains the amount of dental decay which has fallen without a parallel decline in sugar consumption. Decay is not primarily a dietary disease but one of microbial origin. The responsible bacteria form on inadequately cleansed teeth producing acid. These bacteria utilise not just sucrose but much more complex carbohydrates. Even then a crucial factor is how long the teeth remain uncleansed and whether damage is repaired by fluoride. Caries then, like heart disease is multi-factorial with diet a contributing factor and sucrose only part of the linked diet. Thus preventing caries is not easily achieved by simply reducing sucrose intake. Midda lists a number of steps which would further dental health.

8 Obesity: the pleasantly plump should not use the remedies of the highly obese

The most reliable standard of assessing obesity is the ratio of weight to the square of the height of a person. The resulting figures should be allocated to three grades. Grade III are the really fat who will have severe health problems. Treatment is often unsuccessful and life expectancy low. Grade II is also associated with health problems but they can be reduced if weight is lost. This does happen under supervision. Grade I is not associated with major hazards to health. Though those in Grade I do not need to lose weight, they use diets and buy many of the slimming aids. If persons who are pleasantly obese insist on losing weight, they should certainly not use diets suitable for the really obese which need to be administered under medical control. Dr Passmore explains that the current obsession with slimness means that many who should not do so are trying to lose weight often by unsuitable means.

9 Diet and disease: fashions of today and yesterday

Dr James Le Fanu draws attention to the fashionable character of the diet-disease debate. He puts current obsessions with reducing fat intake into perspective by comparison with the advice of the 1930s to increase fat intake. The two sets of advice conflict sharply and both rely on partial and selective interpretation of the available facts. Current advice is not the inevitable result of some recent scientific discovery but reflects the success of self-interested sections of the scientific community in providing messages which mirror society's view of itself.

10 The food-health debate: too much over-simplification

Dr Anthony Leeds spells out some of the lessons to be learned from the way the food-health debate has been conducted. He, like others in *A Diet of Reason* wants distinctions made between individuals and whole populations. Health messages should not be simplified to the point where they misrepresent the research simply in order to make them short and direct enough. Not only will this misinform but it may cause harm. Like Swales, Leeds insists that advice given without knowledge of the person receiving it and their circumstances may encourage him to unhealthy practices. The debate would be better too if contributors made their expertise or lack of it clear, if (financial) interests were declared but not used automatically to discredit contributors, in short if it were a debate committed more to health education and less to mass health propaganda.

11 The methods for changing national diet unlikely to work

Those who argue for a national change of diet involving higher consumption of 'good' and lower consumption of 'bad' foods do not have adequate scientific evidence for the healthiness of the diet they propose or its general applicability but they do at least argue their case. However, when it comes to the methods whereby this new diet would be enforced, they merely assert it. At various times, especially following the NACNE report, it has been proposed that the government intervene in the livestock market to make breeding leaner carcases more rewarding; that the government ban the advertising of 'unhealthy' foods, that it lavishly fund state propaganda on 'healthy eating', that it enforce food product labelling so as to help customers choose their food 'wisely' and even that it tax 'unhealthy goods'. But no evidence has been produced that such policies would, indeed, achieve the ends desired by those who do desire them. It is assumed that because the ends are, at least to their supporters, worthy, there is no need to argue the means.

Yet, as Charles Plouviez points out, many health educators, who are themselves in the advertising business, profoundly misunderstand how and when advertising works and does not work. It is best at increasing a market share for an individual product, much less successful at advocacy. It is doubtful whether it will be of much help in changing national diets, that is in health education campaigns, but it is already of use in providing information about goods which the proposed bans would stop. And regulation in the agricultural market has had precisely the opposite effect to what those who want to lower fat intake desire. Regulation persistently misfires. As Catherine Montgomery Blight and Simon Scanlan remark, 'the higher the incidence of market interference, the less does the resulting product match healthy eating standards'.

One cannot know for certain how the proposed interventions would work but it is surely incumbent on those who advocate them, at considerable public expense and disruption to bring some evidence as to their effects, given the record of other past interventions.

12 The real choice: sensitive, varied knowledge about food and health or state propaganda

The food labelling proposals have the most immediate appeal. At first sight the plea that the customer should be told what is in the tin or packet which he or she is buying seems indeed reasonable. But how much and what sort of information should be given. It would be easy to give a summary of ingredients in scientific terminology but some would-be labellers do not want this. What they want is 'information' which comments on the ingredients, 'information' selected and coded for a purpose, a purpose in the would-be labeller's mind, manipulative labels, labels which explain possible links to health, which are colour-coded to indicate dangers. Such a label is not giving information at all but propaganda. And that is the nub of the whole diet-disease debate. It is not a debate between those who want the public to have more knowledge about food and health and those who don't. It is a debate between those who want the public to have the knowledge as it genuinely is, with all its uncertainties and qualifications, and those who want to issue black and white propaganda which goes well beyond scientific evidence, which ignores differing needs of individuals, which pre-judges scientific inquiries which are currently far from conclusive and which is contemptuous of the ordinary person's ability to assess competing arguments and choose a diet for him or herself and family. The debate is between health educators and 'health' propagandists.

Some propagandists admit, in private, that indeed their case is not conclusive, but, they say, the diet-health problem is so important that we should start the propaganda anyway: it can do no harm; it might do good. That, of course, is a policy decision not a scientific one. It would be better policy if some *policy* evidence were shown supporting it. For the propaganda can do harm. As several contributors have pointed out, eating too little of some foods is as dangerous as eating too much. Firing propaganda at whole nations composed of people eating very different amounts of foods is dangerous. It is dangerous and wrong to pretend to gullible politicians frightened by rising health costs that dietary change offers the nation some sort of easy or cheaper solution to health problems which therapeutic medicine finds daunting: any dietitian knows how difficult it is to get one person to change his diet and that a person the dietitian can talk to face to face and whose circumstances and possible motivations he knows. How much more difficult to 'change the nation's eating habits'.

It is dangerous and wrong to hold out to the man and woman in the street who are still respectful both of scientific research and medicine, hopes of substantially healthier and longer lives for all consequent on their changing their eating, and to do so in the name of science, when science gives no such guarantee. And last, those who would turn advice about food and health into crude propaganda administered by a coercive state give science a bad name. That was the reason most of these contributors gave for wanting to correct current dietary propaganda by contributing to a 'diet of reason'.

2 Dairy Products and Red Meat – Villains or Victims?

Barbara Pickard

1 The popular view – fact or fancy?

From time to time, the in vogue and health-conscious celebrity lets it be known that he shuns red meat and dairy products, and these foods promptly fall further out of favour. Hardly anyone seems to doubt that these traditional constituents of our diet, which for so long have been held in high esteem as superior sources of protein, vitamins and minerals, could suddenly have been transformed from being beneficial to being detrimental to health. Should we really believe that our modern centrally-heated existence has changed our dietary needs substantially or that intensive farming methods have altered these foods out of all recognition, filling them with fat and all manner of other unwanted substances? Or is it mainly that there has been a change in public opinion, a mere following of fashion? Certainly, retailers have jumped on the bandwagon, sensing the profits from 'low fat' and 'active' leisurewear and the health cult devotee of today seems determined not only to inflict his restrictive low-fat vegetarianism and daily jog on himself, but also on anyone within his sphere of influence. Impressionable members of the media quickly spread the message nationwide; television screens depicting scenes of morbid disease juxtaposed with shots of dairy produce and fat meat predictably elicit a pavlovian rejection response. Eventually, the erstwhile 'normal' individual, eating a varied diet and taking moderate but inconspicuous exercise, is scorned for his lack of concern about his health. Dissemination of scientific information and ideas can often result in dilution and obfuscation but in the current diet: health debacle, the reverse seems to have occurred; uncertainties and controversy have been swept aside as being obstructive and reactionary and official recommendations have been sharpened and distorted at each stage of interpretation. The end result of all this is a belief system which is almost totally unrelated to scientific fact; it is the child who when offered a drink of milk refuses on the grounds that it might give him a heart attack; it is the housewife who believes margarine is less fattening than butter and who dare not eat red meat although it might cure her anaemia; it is the middle-aged man who denies himself any visible animal fat, supremely confident that this will insure him against heart disease, and happily oblivious of the insidious undermining of his health caused by his aggressions, frustrations and inability to sleep properly. Even more dangerous, it is those individuals in positions of power, in medicine, politics and the food industry who seem to be forming their opinions from the popular press and television rather than from reasoned scientific publications.

The blame for these warped conceptions of the relationship between health and life-style cannot be placed entirely in the lap of the media; even publications from quasi-scientific bodies such as the Health Education Council lack credibility when making statements about diet. Thus a 1984 publication on pregnancy clearly points out that milk contains fat and too much may lead to high weight gain. Milk is 3.8 per cent fat; the fat in sandwich biscuits (26 per cent), chocolates (30 per cent), and crisps (36 per cent) was not mentioned. Their latest effort *Eating For A Healthier Heart* carries even more indictment of traditional dairy foods and meat: 'The trouble is that some types of milk have a lot of saturated fat in them' and 'The snag [with meat] is the saturated fat that usually comes with it'. Is 2.3 g. of saturated fat in every 100 g. of whole milk really a lot? It also states quite categorically 'Eating too much saturated fat tends to increase the level of cholesterol in the blood, increase the build-up of cholesterol on the inside of the arteries, especially around the heart and increase the risk of a complete blockage, causing a heart attack'. The image of fat congealing in arteries almost as it might on the side of a dinner plate sounds quite credible, especially to the layman. It is not credible at all if one reads in any depth the scientific literature on this subject.

2 The 'official' view – science or compromise?

JACNE states 'The main problem as far as your heart is concerned is too much saturated fat'. Things have come a long way since 1974 when the DHSS committee on medical aspects of food policy concluded that no single dietary factor could be regarded as predominant in determining susceptibility to heart disease. The same view was still prevalent in 1978 when the DHSS book *Eating For Health* recommended a diet which should comprise 'a mixture of many different foods and include cereal foods, protein foods, some fat (to ensure essential fatty acids) and fruit and vegetables'. It did warn of the danger that one particular dietary factor may be taken up with enthusiasm without consideration of other known or suspected risks; a timely prediction in view of events since then. Where does the responsibility lie for this, with the media and those who are not sufficiently informed, or with NACNE, COMA and finally JACNE? The NACNE Report was intended only as a discussion document but soon, thanks to media publicity over alleged attempts to suppress or delay publication, it became the topic of conversation over dinner tables throughout the land. The dairy and meat industries came under particular attack from NACNE, mainly it seemed because of arithmetic simplicity and ease of practical implementation – 'There are obviously many ways in which total fat can be reduced, but some are easier than others to implement...total dairy fat provides about a third of total fat intakes and meat fat approximately 25 per cent. With a reduction in these two sources of fat, the P:S ratio will tend to increase'.

In the wake of NACNE came COMA, the real 'official' view. It recommended that 'consumption of saturated fatty acids and of fat in the UK should be decreased'. It justified its recommendations by referring to 'a more detailed account of evidence...found in the Rationale of the Diet:Heart statement of the American Heart Association'. Yet a review of the original publications on which this statement was based, prompted Reiser to conclude that for the most part, these publications were obsolete or misquoted.

COMA also stated 'Consideration should be given to ways and means of removing from the CAP those elements of it which may discourage individuals and families from implementing the recommendations for dietary change'. The implications for primary producers of food and for suppliers to the agricultural industry were obvious and estimated reductions in the dairy cow herd of 575,000 were envisaged. COMA recommended that 'those responsible for health education should inform the general public of the recommendations and how to implement them'. JACNE sprang into action and produced its leaflet, ostensibly intended as the common man's COMA, though apparently not to the entire satisfaction of the DHSS.

In the decade between the sensible and cautious *Eating for Health* and the JACNE leaflet, had a welter of new research evidence appeared? It would seem not and, if anything, later evidence has merely added further to the confusion. Was it then the result of a demand for consensus and for specific quantitative messages rather than generalities? Consensus is the slogan of the health education movement; consistency of message has come to assume greater importance than the fundamental issue of whether the message is correct. The evidence is by no means as heavyweight as the convictions of the health educators.

3 Evidence from studies between countries not sufficient

COMA's main thrust is based on epidemiology 'Comparisons between countries have shown a strong positive relationship between the proportion of dietary energy derived from saturated fatty acids and mortality from coronary heart disease'. This is not disputed, but do such correlations imply causality? Statistical correlations between various variables should not, of themselves, be considered sufficient evidence of a cause and effect relationship. Children who do not wear shoes are more likely to get malaria; if all children wore shoes, would this eliminate malaria? Even the arch epidemiologists admit that their studies alone cannot decipher which correlations have causal significance and which not. Furthermore, there have been suspicions of biased selection of countries to fit the hypothesis and there has been a blind eye turned to the clear finding that the statistical association of coronary heart disease with milk, meat, saturated fat and total fat is no longer significant when other variables such as smoking and sugar consumption are taken into account.

If one examines the graph showing the simple link between animal fat consumption in countries and coronary heart disease mortality (Figure 1), it is evident that there are two main groupings or clusters; whilst there is a big difference between the two different clusters, within each cluster there is no obvious pattern. Plotting the same data for coronary heart disease deaths against degrees of latitude of the capital city of each country

Figure 1

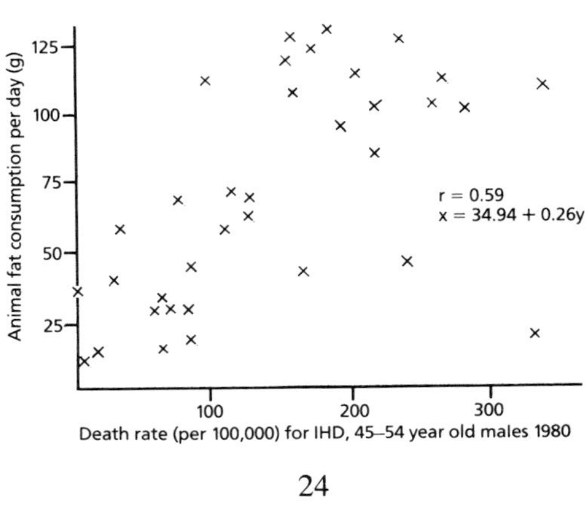

from the equator (Figure 2) also shows a similar relationship. Should we recommend that those wishing to avoid heart disease move closer to the equator?

Figure 2

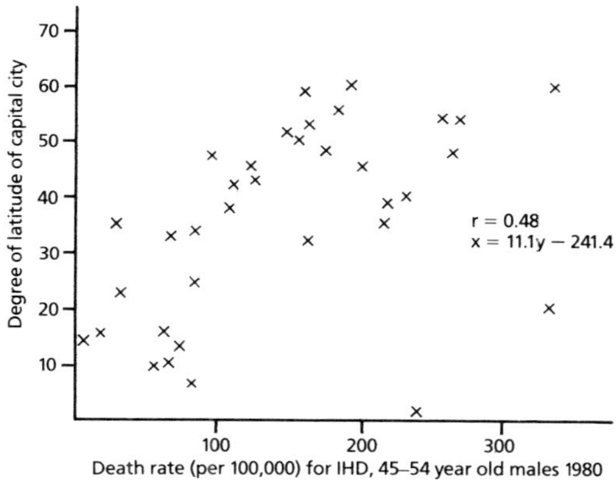

When a comparison is made of the use of red meat and dairy products in the UK compared to the USA and the rest of the EEC, no incriminating pattern appears. The UK consumes less red meat than all the other countries of the EEC which in turn use less than the USA. Red meat available for consumption in the USA in 1982 was 81.4 kg/person/year, 41 per cent more than the comparable figure of 57.8 kg in the UK. Whilst more milk is consumed in the UK than in the USA and in all the EEC countries except Eire, the consumption of butter and cream by the UK (5kg butterfat equivalent/person/year) is well below the 14.6 kg of Denmark and UK cheese consumption, next to the lowest, is a paltry 6.7 kg compared to France's 19.3 kg.

4 Studies within countries inconclusive in causal terms

COMA admitted that within any one country there is no convincing evidence for a relationship between the proportion of dietary energy derived from saturated fatty acids and mortality from coronary heart disease, a statement which is hardly grounds for the clarion calls of the diet evangelists.

Whilst coronary heart disease deaths are becoming commoner in the lower socio-economic groups, there is no significant relationship between the change in heart disease deaths and the change in social class patterns of fat consumption, and geographical comparisons of coronary heart disease incidence within the UK are no more enlightening. Indeed one can select figures for coronary heart disease mortality in nine regions of the UK for 1981 and plot them against total fat as a percentage of total energy intake and find that the trend is quite the opposite of that which one might expect from the current recommendations to reduce total fat to 35 per cent of calories (Figure 3).

Figure 3: Age specific death rates from IHD(410–414)in Males aged 35–44 1981

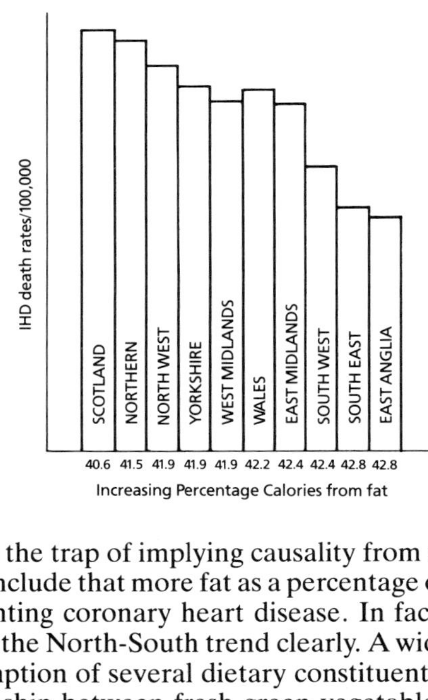

If one fell into the trap of implying causality from such a finding, one might naively conclude that more fat as a percentage of calories might be helpful in preventing coronary heart disease. In fact the national data once again show the North-South trend clearly. A wider investigation of trends in consumption of several dietary constituents revealed a strong negative relationship between fresh green vegetable consumption and coronary heart disease mortality for these same regions, whilst dairy products, meat and butter were not significantly correlated (Figure 4). One might ask why distance from the equator and vegetable consumption have had such a poor press?

In addition to general studies within a country, there have been a number of detailed observational studies on individuals. Of course it

Figure 4: Heart disease mortality and fresh green vegetable consumption.

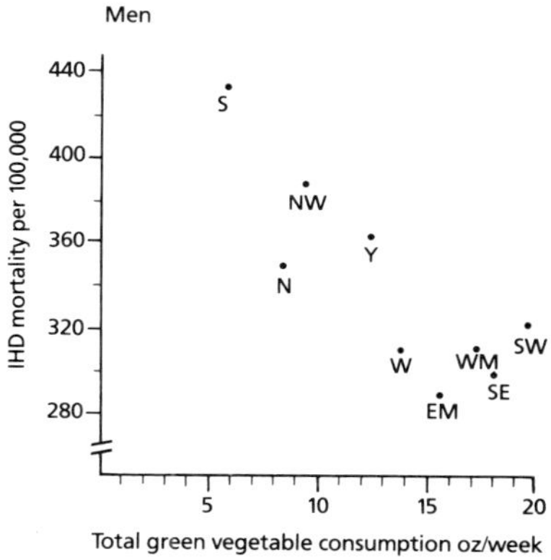

makes obvious sense to find out whether individuals who eat more saturated fat are more at risk than those who consume less. Indeed, this evidence would seem to be a pre-requisite of any dietary advice aimed at individuals, yet this relationship has not been confirmed.

In the Zutphen study in the Netherlands, increases in serum cholesterol over a period of ten years in 871 middle-aged men were not attributable to any change in the percentage of saturated fat in the diet; polyunsaturated fat as a percentage of energy had increased significantly, as also did body weight, despite a decrease in energy intake.

The main findings on energy and fat from five detailed surveys on diet and coronary heart disease are shown in Table 1. The major finding in all the studies was consistent – a negative or inverse relationship between energy intake and coronary heart disease, i.e. those eating more appeared to be less at risk. In some studies, but not all, there were relationships with other factors such as starchy carbohydrate and alcohol, where consumption was higher in men who did not develop heart disease. There was no significant relationship between the amount of fat and saturated fat in the diet and heart disease or between dietary fat and serum cholesterol. However, in some of the trials there was a positive relationship between the percentage of energy derived from fat (both saturated and polyunsaturated) and coronary heart disease incidence. To quote from one report, 'This may be a statistical artifact arising

Table 1: Main Findings of detailed dietary studies on heart disease

Number Of Men	337	859	8,218	7,272	1,994
Nationality	British	American	Puerto Rican	Of Japanese Ancestry	Of Irish Origin
Place	London	Framingham	San Juan	Honolulu	Boston/Ireland
Any significant relation of CHD with:–					
Total amount of fat?	No	No	No	No	No
Amount of saturated fat?	No	No	No	No	No
Energy intake?*	Yes	Yes	Yes	Yes	Yes
Other factors?*	Fibre	Alcohol	Starch	Starch	Unrefined Carbohydrate

* Negative correlation; i.e. increased consumption associated with lower CHD risk.

from their lower calorie intake. When the level of these nutrients is expressed in absolute terms, it bears no relation to coronary heart disease risk'. Is then much of the current advice on percentage of fat in the diet based on a 'statistical artifact'?

In a recent twenty-year follow-up of the Irish-based study which was shown in Table 1, there were no significant differences in the age-adjusted mean percentages of animal fat, saturated fat or total fat between those who died of coronary heart disease and those who did not. By complex statistical manipulations, the authors were able to suggest in the abstract that those who died may have had a relatively higher intake of saturated fat and cholesterol and lower polyunsaturated fatty acid consumption . However, in the main text of the article there was less conviction – 'The nature of the association in this study between dietary lipids and the risk of mortality from coronary heart disease remains unclear. As intake increases, one expects the risk to increase or decrease steadily. However, this did not always happen'. Indeed those individuals who were in the middle had the lowest risk of death of all; in other words subjects on moderate intakes were less at risk than those who ate *less* fat as well as those who ate more. The authors commented on the trends in coronary heart disease mortality 'The changes in dietary levels of complex carbohydrates match the risk more closely than the changes in dietary lipid levels'. Indeed examination of the raw data showed that the vegetable food score was more highly significant than other dietary variables – the more vegetables eaten, the less the risk of coronary heart disease. The authors gave more examples of evidence to support a protective role for vegetable foods in the prevention of coronary heart disease. Again fat might merely be a marker for the disease; increasing fat could be indirectly involved insofar as excess fat must mean less of some other dietary constituents such as vegetables and cereals which may be protective.

5 Trends in animal fat consumption over time not causally related
Changes in diet over time, either for the 'worse' or 'better', are often claimed to result in increases or declines in coronary heart disease mortality rates. Indeed the JACNE booklet states 'In countries like the USA where people have made changes, deaths from heart disease are now much less common and are still decreasing .... Food, especially the amount of *fat* in your food, has an important part to play in this change'. Can this view be upheld by available evidence?

In the USA there was an obvious decline in recorded coronary heart disease deaths from 1968 to 1975. During this period fat in the food supply was still rising to peak in 1972; the increase being attributable mainly to vegetable sources; the decline in animal fat consumption was however only a few grams per day and saturated fat as a percentage of total calories changed little at around 15 per cent. In fact animal fat as a proportion of total fat in the food supply had been declining since the turn of the century. In 1967 to 1969 dairy products (excluding butter) supplied 12.3 per cent of fat and in 1982 11.7 per cent; meat, poultry and fish supplied 37.3 per cent in 1967 to 1969 and 34.0 per cent in 1982; hardly a massive decline over that period. Butter continued its downward trend too.

Table 2: Fat In The American Food Supply

	Total Fat	*Animal Fat*		*Vegetable Fat*		*Saturated Fat*		
	g/day	*g/day*	*%*	*g/day*	*%*	*g/day*	*% of total*	*% of calories*
1909–13	126	105	83	21	17	49.8	40	13
1965	144	95	66	49	34	53.9	37	15.3
1976	157	89	57	68	43			
1982	162	92	57	70	43	54.1	33	14

So what did change, if anything, in the American diet over this period? Between 1967–9 and 1982 the largest gain was for ascorbic acid (vitamin C), due to increased use of citrus fruits and dark green or deep yellow vegetables. Diets deficient in vegetables and vitamin C have both been implicated at various times in relation to heart disease.

A similar pattern of fat intake has emerged from studies of dietary change in this country. The proportion of fat coming from animal sources has declined whilst that from vegetable sources has increased (Figure 5).

Figure 5: Proportions of fat from animal and vegetable sources

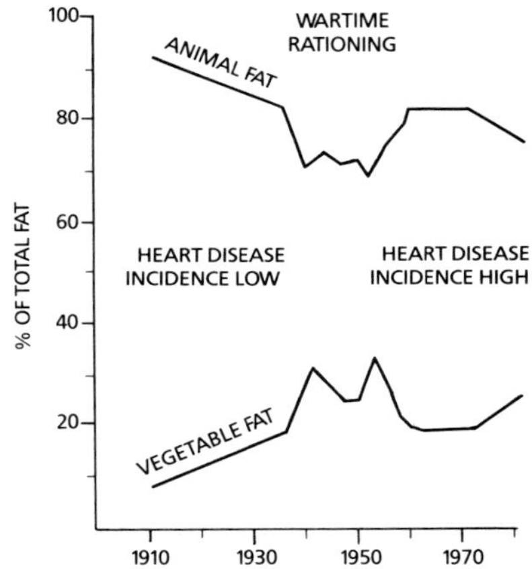

The oft-quoted reduction in coronary heart disease mortality in war-time on a controlled diet takes no account of the fact that dietary changes caused by rationing continued well into the 1950s when coronary heart disease rates were again on the increase. Food supply data for the UK show that meat and dairy products (excluding butter), together contributed 61 per cent of total fat in 1909–13 and declined to 49 per cent by 1962, and estimates for 1981 showed that these two food groups contributed together 46 per cent of total fat in the diet of households surveyed in 1981. This latter is a consumption estimate and is not dissimilar from consumption estimates from the US survey in 1977–8.

Table 3: Fat Consumption In 1981: U.K. And The U.S.A. 1977–8

	Fat Consumption g/day		*Fat Consumption as a % of total fat*	
	U.K.	*U.S.A.*	*U.K.*	*U.S.A.*
Dairy	19.5	13.9	18.9	16.8
Meat	28.0	35.1	27.0	42.4
Dairy + Meat	47.5	49.0	45.9	59.2
Total Fat	89.9	82.8		

Between 1959 and 1972 when coronary heart disease mortality in men was increasing, in the UK the average consumption of saturated fat remained stationary, whilst polyunsaturated fat increased by 25 per cent. From 1979 to 1982, when the fall in coronary heart disease mortality for men aged 45 to 54 in England and Wales was greater than that seen in the USA from 1968 to 1975, saturated fat consumption fell a mere 3.4g. per day.

Not only do the UK and USA not give any clear indication of a concurrent relationship between diet and coronary heart disease mortality; trends in other countries similarly do not show any obvious pattern. Examination of dietary change from 1947 to 1962 and changes in coronary heart disease mortality from 1955 to 1965 in 37 countries led Masironi to conclude that there was no obvious link with any particular dietary constituent. Indeed his data showed that the countries which had the most dramatic rise in coronary heart disease mortality (Poland and Yugoslavia) had experienced the largest decline in saturated fat consumption; on the other hand, Switzerland, which had increased its consumption of total fat and of saturated fat had the largest decline in coronary heart disease mortality.

There is thus no obvious link between dietary change over time and coronary heart disease mortality but some have argued that this is because of misinterpretations. One argument presented is that food supply data do not reflect consumption patterns. Certainly this is particularly obvious for the USA, where food supply estimates for total fat were 161 g./person/day whilst consumption surveys estimated total fat eaten to be more in the region of 83 g./person/day. Even with an estimated fat waste of 40 g./day (including fat waste from dairy products and table spreads, estimated at less than one gram per day, and from meat, poultry and fish, 29 g. per day, etc.), there is still a large amount to be accounted for. These discrepancies illustrate the great difficulty of assessing actual fat consumed and also in reaching realistic conclusions as to its causal significance, if any. Surveys of actual consumption are themselves not very precise and are rendered even more difficult to evaluate because of their omissions. For example the National Household Food Survey in the UK is derived from foods entering households but does not include alcohol, sweets or chocolates, nor does it make full allowance for food eaten outside the home. Nevertheless the differences in the UK data between fat in the food supply (128 g./day for 1982) and fat consumed (103 g./day) are not so large as in the USA. Whether data from the food supply or from consumption estimates are used, they are useful in showing trends over time but there is no clear relationship of coronary heart disease mortality with particular elements of diet. Total fat in the American diet from consumption estimates is still 42 per cent of calories.

Another argument by the diet lobby is that changes in coronary heart disease mortality over time cannot be reflected by contemporary changes in diet because the development of coronary heart disease involves a latent period. Phillip Burch, in his study of risk factors and coronary heart disease, estimated the latent periods to average 10 years for men and 20 for women and reported that trends in mortality did not reflect dietary trends even when latency periods were taken into account.

6 Dietary advice for the population – inappropriate for the individual?
The blanket recommendations about diet which are being made are intended for more or less all except the under-fives. These recommendations, whilst perhaps not inappropriate for the hypercholesterolaemic middle-aged overweight underactive executive accustomed to rich food, may not be of benefit to others and could even be harmful to some, such as growing children, active adults and women contemplating pregnancy as well as those already pregnant or breastfeeding.

Despite a glut of EEC surpluses, many young women in this country may be under-nourished, some for cosmetic reasons, others because of poverty. A below-normal weight for height before pregnancy, coupled with poor weight gain during pregnancy, is a very good recipe for producing a low birth-weight child; a child more likely to be mentally and physically behind its heavier equivalent for many years if not for life. The proportion of babies in the UK which are in the low birth-weight category is still too high, more than one in every 14 babies. Detailed studies on the diets of pregnant women of low socio-economic status have indicated that under-nourishment of the mother was a likely cause of low birth-weight. The women were eating significantly fewer calories and significantly less fat, both saturated and polyunsaturated, than pregnant women in higher socio-economic groups, who were giving birth to heavier babies. What price a low-fat diet to impoverished pregnant women?

Although COMA excluded children under five from their recommendations and JACNE excluded 'infants', professionals in the Health Service as well as diet-conscious parents may not all heed this advice. Children have a relatively greater energy requirement than adults for growth and development as well as for activity. Also they can less easily cope with the large volumes of low-calorie foods which high fibre low-fat diets often entail. Meat and milk, on the other hand, are easily digestible foods which contain high quality protein as well as minerals such as iron, zinc and calcium. Dairy products are the major source of calcium in the diet whilst the 'haem' iron in meat is much better absorbed than non-haem iron from non-animal sources. Not only is zinc better absorbed from animal than vegetable sources, but also the zinc content of 100 calories-worth of beef brisket is twice that of the equivalent calorie serving of chicken, lentils or beans.

Even in 1970, one in 10 of 10-year old children surveyed in the National Child Development survey stated they hardly ever ate meat and one in five only ate meat 'sometimes'. The emerging picture is that children in the lower socio-economic groups are less likely to be eating meat and cheese but more likely to be consuming confectionery and soft drinks, expensive but much less nutritious alternatives. Whole milk consumption too has been falling, especially in the younger age groups and this fall has not been entirely offset by increased intakes of skimmed milk, perhaps partly because of the inferior taste and poor keeping quality of skimmed milk, but also because of increased soft drink consumption. Milk consumption in two-to-nine-year olds fell 25 per cent from 1.6 litres per person per week in 1970–1 to 1.2 litres in 1980–1, whilst soft drink consumption increased 40 per cent from 1.85 litres to 2.6 litres per person per week. A similar trend occurred in other age groups, except the over 65s. For many children then, meat and dairy products are being replaced by ever more highly-refined snacks and drinks, often containing little but calories and colour. It is even possible that some parents consider that this trend away from meat and dairy foods has official approval.

The anomaly is that whilst whole milk may have the popular veto if you want to avoid a heart attack, it has the go-ahead for protecting against some forms of cancer, as described in the recent report on diet and cancer from the American National Academy of Sciences. Another example is that of the fashionable female taking strenuous exercise; she is going to increase her need for the vitamin riboflavin, the main source of this being dairy products, paradoxically something she is quite likely to be avoiding.

Recent evidence suggests that calcium has an important role to play in relation to blood pressure; low calcium intakes are linked with a greater incidence of hypertension. The recent report of a 50-year old American businessman with hypertension is yet another case of dietary fashion being carried to extremes. This man, until a few years beforehand in excellent health, experienced an increased blood pressure which drug therapy failed to cure (although drug use was linked with weight gain, sexual dysfunction, exercise intolerance, and inability to concentrate). After months of ineffective treatment, he decided to seek a second opinion, and it was discovered that because of fear of heart disease, he had for the previous few years virtually abstained from all milk and cheese. He was advised to liberalise his diet to include more dairy produce and achieve an intake of one gram of calcium daily. Within two weeks his blood pressure was normal; drugs were then discontinued and over the next six weeks all other side effects disappeared. The author of the report, Dr McCarron, commented 'It is thus important for physicians to realise, in our present state of ignorance about the causation of the major chronic disorders, that variety and moderation in diet is the best advice for all reasonably healthy persons. Imbalances can be caused by over-zealous practices of dietary restriction which adversely affect the overall health of the individual'.

7 Focus on animal fat and serum cholesterol ignores other dietary constituents

It is a puzzling feature of the whole debate that whilst the proponents of the saturated fat:high blood cholesterol:heart disease theory can produce evidence in support of their argument for whole nations or even for large groups, on an individual basis the relationship does not seem to hold true. An individual's serum cholesterol level seems to be controlled by some homeostatic mechanism which is little influenced by diet. The level can change but dietary fat, including beef fat and dairy fat, does not seem to be any more likely, or even as likely, to affect it as all manner of other things, such as genetics, cultural tradition, exercise, anxiety, or even low temperature. Furthermore, a diet change which may result in a fall in serum cholesterol in one individual may cause an increase in another.

Even in experiments or intervention trials where a mean overall response of serum cholesterol to dietary change has been demonstrated, the response is often small and its effect on heart disease unknown. Claims that the change was due to a change in the amount and type of fat consumed frequently ignore that other changes in diet and lifestyle have also been made. If an experiment is carried out in which variables A, B, C, D and E are changed and an effect is seen, is it good science to conclude that the result was a direct effect of a change in A, rather than B, C, D or even all of them? In a detailed study of some families in North Karelia, the part of Finland which wages an active campaign against coronary heart disease, there was a 28 per cent reduction in smoking, a change to a diet low in fat with a high P:S ratio, an overall decline in energy intake, increased consumption of vegetables and fruit with a significant increase in the intake of vitamin C. The resultant statistically significant fall in serum cholesterol may receive publicity in relation to changes in the fat in the diet but it could well have been affected by any or all of the other variables. Lower calorie intake can result in a lowering of serum cholesterol as too may a cessation of smoking. The vitamin/mineral content of the diet could have been relevant; certainly vitamin C deficiency appears to be linked with high levels of blood cholesterol and deficiencies of other vitamins and minerals such as magnesium and calcium have been implicated. Recently, there have been suggestions that vegetable foods could modify risk by lowering blood pressure or serum cholesterol. These are surely factors worthy of further investigation in the UK especially since it sits bottom of the league table in terms of vitamin C consumption and it is well known that fresh vegetable consumption in Scotland falls below that of England and Wales, whereas coronary heart disease mortality is higher.

Whilst COMA made no specific recommendations about the intake of oxidised cholesterol, it did advocate more research to ascertain whether it may be involved in atherosclerosis. This would certainly seem to be a pressing topic for research, as pointed out in a recent review; auto-oxidation products of cholesterol have been found in highly processed foods such as instant mixes and concentrated infant formulas.

8 Other damaging effects of the accepted dogma

A great deal of harm could be done to the prospects for future research on coronary heart disease. The common assumption that the cause has been identified may divert attention and much-needed funds away from worthy research projects. These include studies on other dietary constituents and on non-dietary variables such as behavioural traits, sleep patterns, genetics, and traditional patterns of culture. For example, much attention has been paid to the low incidence of coronary heart disease in Japan and the increase in incidence which occurs when Japanese migrate to America; yet one research study showed that Japanese in America who ate a western diet but retained their Japanese culture of upbringing had a lower prevalence of coronary heart disease than Japanese there who were eating a Japanese diet, whether or not they adopted a traditional or non-traditional culture. The non-traditional culture group as a whole were by far the worst with reference to coronary heart disease, whether aged under 45 or 45–54.

Failure to encourage research to investigate these issues further will not only have repercussions on the scientists directly involved but also ultimately on the rest of the medical profession. As the 'anti-fat' fad passes into the realms of history, as did the fashions against bread and potatoes, it is not unlikely that those false prophets in health education and medicine, and many others too, will lose credibility in the eyes of the general public. Whilst this may be no bad thing for matters controversial, it could easily result in a failure to follow advice in relation to issues where there is stronger evidence, such as smoking.

Another area of concern has to do with the growing spectre of legislation and regulations on diet. If the diet evangelists have their way, such bureaucratic threats may become reality, regardless of the weakness of the scientific evidence. Furthermore, those critical of restrictions of individual freedom in other countries would do well to focus attention on the insidious development in this country of propaganda-type broadcasting on dietary issues. It is astonishing that the deliberations of TV and radio producers and presenters are more influential than those of full-time professionals working on diet and disease.

The effect which so few can have on so many is not just related to what is on the menu in a household tomorrow or next year; it has to do with the whole framework of society. Unnecessary damage will be done to the agricultural industry, especially to the livestock industry. Puzzled milk producers, still staggering from the imposition of quota restrictions by the EEC, now face even further economic hardships as a result of falling consumption, and many suffer needless remorse that their produce may have been harming the health of the nation. Meat producers, after working for years to develop systems of livestock management to try and put fat on animals have to learn to cater instead for the latest demand for lean meat. After investing heavily to produce more and more, the farmer may now be saddled with a lifetime burden of debt, a debt which government actively encouraged him to take on. Industries which depend on the livestock industry, such as machinery manufacturers and suppliers of animal feeds, all face cutbacks too.

The man in the street may not have the rug of his livelihood pulled from under his feet but he has a price to pay. Does he not feel a sense of guilt if he dares to enjoy cream on his fruit, a nice wedge of traditional cheddar or the fat-trim on his meat? His paranoia about food is accentuated by the dismal feeling that he and he alone is responsible for whether he gets a heart attack or not. This burden of responsibility is totally out of context to the evidence. At the other end of the scale is the devoted follower of the prudent diet:exercise regime who is left struggling to understand how or why he ended up in a coronary care unit.

The general air of pessimism which abounds today about heart disease is oddly not related to the pattern of coronary heart disease mortality. Little attention was focussed on it while the death rate was rising but now that it is falling, there is a sudden upsurge of interest. Whilst numbers of people affected are increasing as we proceed towards a society top heavy with the older age groups, there is overall an age-related decline. Indeed Burch calculated that the rate of fall in England and Wales from 1979–83 for men aged 45–54 was larger than that for US whites from 1968–75. This is not widely known, nor is the point which COMA made that 'most deaths from cardiovascular disease occur in old age, the median age of death being 74 years for coronary heart disease'. Whilst coronary heart disease deaths exceed those due to other causes, this is partly because of a decline in deaths from other causes such as infection.

9 Conclusions

The die has been cast and animal fat will have to suffer the consequences for the next few years at least. While those in discourse in corners of academia may fervently condemn the current in-vogue hypothesis, there will be but few who dare to stir the waters of consensus. Indeed there are few who remain free to do so; perhaps the occasional academic with time to spare, the critical and questioning general practitioner or the interested cardiologist. Of the rest, a large proportion have their hands already tied, some suffer from the 'little bit of knowledge is a dangerous thing' syndrome, and many more just do not want to get involved. The dissenting NHS dietitian can hardly stand up and condemn the local NHS food policy; the home economist must adhere to the latest curriculum changes; and the nutritionist in industry does not want to ruffle the feathers of the establishment. Whilst those involved in selling products which can be labelled 'low fat' or 'high in polyunsaturates' can sit back and wallow in all the free advertising, those who try to market meat, milk and cheese have opted to restrain themselves from confronting the fundamental issues and, unable to bury their heads in the sand instead, busy themselves with indirect prattle. Perhaps they suffer from committee disease and their considered opinion depends on those voting members whose opinions are swayed by the daily paper rather than by the research paper.

Certainly committee disease is a major problem. As Professor Mitchell pointed out 'The claim that the collective beliefs of a prestigious committee can provide a substitute for facts is all too prevalent;...Unfortunately, just as we cannot be sure of the relationship between risk factors and disease, we cannot be sure of the relationship between the opinion of the committee and the truth; the opinion of the committee will depend on who is selected for it'. Members of these committees appear to come to different conclusions depending on whether they wear the hat of a policy-maker or that of a scientist. Science may suggest that the evidence is woolly and uncertain; that it may be better to throw out the theory and try again; politics and policy-making demand certain statements and no sitting on the fence; better to throw out the evidence. Maybe too in the final analysis the plethora of research papers on this subject has not been beneficial; for those who are bidden to produce a review paper, it is easier to rely on abstracts and summaries rather than attempt the mammoth task of critical examination of methods and main text. Differences which require a statistical microscope to detect may well have little practical or biological relevance but findings which are uncertain in the text can become translated into generalities in the abstract, into the new certainties in the review and soon become 'fact' to the general public.

Change is unlikely whilst the current power struggle is in the court of those in the food industry who are likely to benefit from the thumbs down on red meat and dairy products. After all, the surplus funds available for campaigning by the Milk Marketing Board and the Meat and Livestock Commission are nothing in comparison. Is the lack of financial strength of the fresh vegetable lobby one possible reason for its apparent failure to be brought into the public eye? If consensus were needed amongst professionals, surely it would be achieved over the benefits of fresh vegetables as part of a mixed diet, yet vegetables have had few bouquets. The reason one might suspect is financial, there being no massively organised and wealthy industry to back up those who grow, transport and market these commodities.

If the recommendations on diet had been to eat a wide range of foods and to include among them those which are fresh such as fruit and vegetables, and those which are basic staples such as milk and dairy produce, bread and cereals, together with meat, fish, poultry and eggs, the health of the nation might well have benefited. It is worthy of note that there is increased interest in fresh and perishable groceries in the supermarkets of North America, 'dry' groceries appear to be falling out of favour. How long will we be left behind by the 'official' obsession with saturated fat?

Notes and References

B.M. Pickard, 'The CAP, food policy and human health' in D.B. Ross (ed.), *The Effects of the EEC Common Agricultural Policy on Animal Production and Veterinary Medicine*, Proceedings of the Symposium of the Association of Vets in Industry October 1985, Royal College of Veterinary Surgeons, 1986.

B.M. Pickard, 'A counter-review to the COMA report', paper given at the Annual General Meeting of the Society of Feed Technologists, April 1986.

3 Diet and Heart Disease: Mass Interventions or Individualised Treatments?

Donald J. McNamara

1 The confusing debate about fats and heart disease

The rationale for dietary recommendations to the general public in an attempt to reduce the incidence of cardiovascular diseases in industrialised societies has been extensively debated in the scientific literature and public press. One side in the debate recommends that everyone, including children over the ages of two to five years, reduce the intake of total fat, specifically saturated animal fats, and cholesterol in the diet. Dietary recommendations are made in the belief that the specific dietary changes will reduce blood cholesterol levels and in theory will reduce the population's risks of coronary heart disease. In contrast, the antagonists of generalised dietary recommendations question the efficacy of dietary interventions in reducing plasma cholesterol levels and heart disease risk, and support greater effort towards individualised approaches to the treatment of the multifactorial risk factors for heart disease. Differences in opinions on the theoretical benefits from mass dietary interventions are further complicated by the substantially different dietary recommendations and guidelines being proposed by various health professionals on both sides of the Atlantic. Unfortunately, one effect of this debate is a confused public faced with a baffling array of dietary suggestions and constant exposure to the protagonists and antagonists of generalised dietary recommendations.

2 What the individual consumer of food wants to know

What the individual patient really wants is a clear answer to the following questions. Who should I listen to and believe? Which diet should I follow? Am I at risk from heart disease? How can I, or do I need to, reduce my blood cholesterol level? How should I reduce my overall heart disease risk profile? It is not surprising that the public is both confused and apprehensive about the role of diet in overall health and that many people are developing a 'good food – bad food' mentality. Such attitudes towards the role of diet in health can lead to exclusion of some of the highest quality nutrients in the basic diet. Overall nutritional quality, balance and moderation, and the four food groups have been replaced by an attitude that certain foods cause disease while other foods prevent disease, and that what one eats, rather than supplying nutrients and being one of life's pleasures, is a major determinant of the cause of one's mortality.

This chapter attempts to address the role of diet in the cause and prevention of heart disease and the extent to which success might be achieved, in terms of risk reduction, by population-wide changes in the diet. It will also address the relative benefits of public intervention versus individualized approaches to heart disease risk factor reduction. Since there are at least two recommended diets of significance, the more stringent diet recommended by the American Heart Association (AHA) and the modest intervention proposed by the British Committee on the Medical Aspects of Food Policy (COMA) Commission, this essay will address the more drastic AHA diet since it not only recommends the greatest change but in theory should provide the most benefit in terms of a reduction in heart disease incidence.

3 A link between fat and cholesterol but which fats, for which patients and what sort of link?

Epidemiological studies provide the strongest evidence for a relationship among dietary cholesterol and saturated fat, as percent of total calories, an elevated blood cholesterol level and an increased incidence of heart disease. These epidemiological studies do not, however, provide evidence that changing the dietary consumption of cholesterol and saturated animal fats will reduce heart disease incidence. There exist numerous dietary and life-style variables between populations with differing heart disease mortality rates and a direct cause and effect relationship between single components of the diet and heart disease incidence cannot be unequivocally established.

In support of the epidemiological evidence for a relationship between diet and plasma cholesterol levels, controlled metabolic studies in hospital wards have shown that shifting the quality of dietary fat from a low to high polyunsaturated to saturated (P/S) fat ratio reduces plasma cholesterol levels in the majority of patients. The observed reductions vary substantially from patient to patient depending upon the individual's sensitivity to dietary fat; however, a high P/S fat diet will usually reduce plasma cholesterol levels in the majority of patients. Recent studies have shown that monounsaturated fat, such as found in olive oil, also has plasma cholesterol-lowering capabilities in man. The concept that dietary polyunsaturated and monounsaturated fats lower while saturated fats raise plasma cholesterol levels cannot be considered a scientific dogma however. Recent reports have shown that beef fat, classified as saturated and hence hypercholesterolemic, has almost the same lowering effects on plasma cholesterol levels as polyunsaturated safflower oil. Nutritionists and dietitians are faced with the quandary of not being certain which fats elevate and which fats reduce plasma cholesterol levels nor precisely which dietary fat changes should be recommended to the individual patient. There is little doubt that dietary fat quality affects plasma cholesterol levels; what is becoming increasingly more confusing is which fats have what effects and whether modest changes in dietary fat P/S ratio, as recommended, will significantly reduce plasma cholesterol levels in the majority of the population.

The debate over the effects of dietary cholesterol on plasma cholesterol levels is even more confusing since dietary cholesterol and saturated fats are usually ingested together in most animal-derived foods. Controlled metabolic cholesterol feeding studies in hospitals are at variance with the large numbers of outpatient studies carried out feeding low and high cholesterol diets, often by adding eggs to the basal low-cholesterol diet. The evidence for an effect of dietary cholesterol on plasma cholesterol levels was judged insufficient by COMA which did not recommend that the public reduce dietary cholesterol intake. In contrast, the AHA judged the evidence strong enough to make a reduction in dietary cholesterol intake part of the implementation of a 'prudent diet'.

The questions addressed in this essay are whether or not a reduction in dietary cholesterol and saturated fat intake should be expected to:

1) Reduce plasma cholesterol levels in the population.
2) Reduce heart disease incidence.
3) Be free of any side effects or overall nutritional risks.

4 Will a fat-modified diet reduce plasma cholesterol levels?

There is little doubt that dietary fat, both its quality and quantity, and dietary cholesterol affect plasma cholesterol levels. The question under discussion is whether the recommended dietary changes will significantly reduce plasma cholesterol levels in the majority of the population. Two aspects of the evidence for such dietary changes are controversial: the comparison of drastic dietary shifts which have been shown to be effective plasma-cholesterol-lowering interventions as compared to the more modest dietary changes recommended by health organisations; and the large degree of heterogeneity of plasma cholesterol responses seen in patients placed on similar fat-modified diets.

There is little debate that a dietary change from a lard based diet (P/S 0.2) to a corn oil diet (P/S 4.5) will lower plasma cholesterol in most individuals; however, changes from the current diet with a P/S ratio of 0.45 to the recommended 1.0 would not be expected to exert as substantial a reduction in plasma lipid levels. Even in controlled metabolic studies it has been shown that similar moderate shifts in dietary fat quality fail to significantly reduce plasma cholesterol levels in a large number of study subjects. The severely hyperlipidemic patient may well change his or her diet to a more 'prudent' one, yet if the clinician is not aware of the patient's response to the shift in diet and the diet's efficacy, or lack of, as a plasma-cholesterol-lowering intervention, then who will decide which patients require drug interventions to lower their risk of heart disease or who may possibly benefit from other types of dietary interventions.

The question of whether or not dietary cholesterol significantly influences plasma cholesterol levels is equally controversial. Controlled metabolic trials indicate that humans are sensitive to dietary cholesterol and that intake of a high cholesterol diet results in higher plasma cholesterol levels. In contrast, numerous studies in patients fed solid food diets with and without added eggs indicate that humans have relatively precise abilities to compensate for a moderate dietary cholesterol intake. Since the body's own production of cholesterol (~ 700 mg/day) is substantially greater than what most individuals absorb from their diets (~ 250 mg/day), it is not surprising that the body's various control mechanisms can function to keep plasma cholesterol levels constant when dietary cholesterol varies over a modest range of intakes.

There also exist the problems of how well and who will educate the public to make effective dietary changes, particularly on a population-wide basis where nutrition education is so lacking. Most people equate plasma cholesterol with dietary cholesterol and their first, and often only, approach to a dietary change is to exclude foods containing cholesterol from their diet, especially eggs. Many also make ineffectual changes based on the cholesterol content of food stuffs and not on the dietary fat quality. Substituting hydrogenated saturated vegetable oil for animal fat because it has no cholesterol has little effect on plasma cholesterol levels and leaves the individual patient with the misconception that he has changed his diet to a more healthy one when in fact he may well remain at his original risk from heart disease.

Can dietary changes lower the plasma cholesterol levels of the population? Probably to a small extent on a population-wide basis; to such a small extent that the individual with an elevated plasma cholesterol level, who really needs to reduce that level, will remain at an increased risk of developing heart disease. Numerous studies have shown a great heterogeneity of sensitivities to dietary fat and cholesterol when individual patients are considered; the mean response may be a reduction in the average plasma cholesterol level but on an individual basis it is impossible to predict how a given patient may respond to a dietary change. Without diagnosis of hyperlipidemia and follow up evaluation and treatment, the at-risk patient wanders in a maze of dietary changes with the prospect of gaining little benefit. But the argument can be raised that the majority of the population would achieve some reduction in plasma cholesterol levels and therefore in heart disease incidence by changing from a high animal fat and cholesterol intake, and isn't it reasonable to recommend dietary changes for everyone so that some people will benefit?

5 Will a fat-modified diet reduce the incidence of heart disease?

Two questions address the basis of the debate regarding the advisability of dietary recommendations to the general public. Who is at risk from heart disease due to an elevated plasma cholesterol level? Will heart disease incidence be reduced by lowering plasma cholesterol levels with dietary interventions? The best evidence for a relationship between plasma cholesterol levels and heart disease risk comes from epidemiological and population studies such as the National Cooperative Pooling Project. The Pooling Project data indicated that an increased risk of heart disease is clearly apparent once plasma cholesterol levels reach 240 mg/dl. Below this cholesterol level there is little gradation in the risk profile. The data have been interpreted by some to indicate that a threshold exists for the relationship between plasma cholesterol levels and heart disease risk with risk increasing in subjects as cholesterol levels increase beyond 240 mg/dl. Although there is considerable debate on the actual plasma cholesterol level at which heart disease risk begins to accelerate, the Pooling Project data provide the best available evidence we have to date.

Let us assume for the sake of argument that initiation of a fat-modified diet could achieve a five per cent lowering of plasma cholesterol levels. (I pick five per cent because that is the best that has been accomplished in the clinical trials carried out to date; clinical trials where the subjects receive counselling and follow-up by a trained dietitian.) For the high risk patient with an initial cholesterol level of 275 mg/dl the benefit of a dietary change would be a post-intervention cholesterol level of 261 mg/dl and the patient remains at high risk from heart disease. Similarly, for the average male with a cholesterol level of 210 mg/dl we achieve a diet mediated reduction to 200 mg/dl resulting in no appreciable change in heart disease risk. The question rarely addressed in discussions of dietary recommendations is who will benefit from a change in dietary fat and cholesterol. It would appear that those at high risk gain little benefit while the average 'normocholesterolemic' individual is not at risk to start with since his plasma cholesterol is not in the risk region. The best estimates would suggest that those at moderate risk due to a slightly elevated plasma cholesterol level and those exhibiting a high sensitivity to dietary fat and cholesterol would gain some risk reduction from a dietary change. Yet here we are faced with the uncertainty of knowing what proportion of the population falls into any category of expected responses.

6 Are fat-modified diets nutritionally safe?

Animal products in the diet provide a number of essential nutrients and it seems unjustified to give the public the impression that these valuable foodstuffs are hazardous to their health. Implementation of such attitudes runs the risk of imbalancing the overall nutritional pattern of dietary zealots. Calcium is required for bone development and maintenance and the principal source is dairy products, one of the perceived 'bad foods'. Iron needs are met primarily from red meats which also provide high-quality protein and many other important nutrients. Eggs, the knave of the diet-heart disease debate, have become almost *verboten* in a health-conscious diet yet provide high quality nutrition at a reasonable cost, possess cooking qualities which are important in so many enjoyable foods and, in the case of the elderly, are easy to cook, chew and digest. Does it make good sense to exclude or limit these valuable foods from the diets of every man, woman, and child in the hope that plasma cholesterol levels and heart disease incidence may be reduced.

Perhaps the real risk of the recommended fat-modified diet doesn't reside in its nutritional quality, which can be balanced if patients are taught to make effective changes, as much as in its potential to give a false sense of effective risk reduction. Imagine an adult male, 30 pounds overweight, watching his football game on a Saturday afternoon with his blood pressure pounding at 150 over 100 and already starting his second pack of cigarettes while his spouse is in the kitchen preparing his fat-modified dinner. Or on the other hand imagine the patient who really does wish to reduce his risk factors for heart disease, makes effective changes in his diet but unfortunately is relatively diet insensitive, remains at high risk due to an elevated plasma cholesterol and is not being treated by a physician who could initiate cholesterol lowering medication. In both cases, more so in the first than in the second, it is probable that little risk reduction has been achieved by dietary intervention.

7 Is it for individuals or populations to change their diet?

There are a number of dietary factors which influence plasma cholesterol levels to varying degrees in different patients: monounsaturated fats, low total fat intakes, high polyunsaturated fat intakes, dietary fibre, etc. Should we really expect a single 'prudent diet' to be equally beneficial for all patients or wouldn't it make more sense to try different dietary interventions in the treatment of the high risk patient to find the most effective intervention for that patient? A single 'magic bullet' diet is neither universally effective nor a reasonable approach to risk factor reduction when faced with the variability to be found in an individual patient.

Multiple risk factor intervention in the individual patient, as opposed to dietary management in the population, has a number of clear benefits: feedback to the patient since he or she is being monitored; evaluation of the efficacy of any intervention and modification of that intervention to fit the patient's lifestyle; and the clinical determination of whether pharmacological treatment of hypercholesterolemia is required to reduce what may be a non-responsive risk factor.

There are a number of genetic disorders which have been shown to be related to an increased risk of heart disease and no doubt a number of others yet to be discovered. Dietary interventions for these disorders are discouragingly ineffective and more severe measures for risk intervention are required. Without diagnosis and initiation of specific therapy these patients cannot reduce their risk profile and will gain little from dietary changes. With emphasis primarily on population-wide diet-mediated risk factor intervention, those patients who are clearly at elevated risk will be neither diagnosed nor treated appropriately.

8 What are the lessons for public health policy?

Heart disease is a multifactorial disease for which some, but not all, of the risk factors are known. The three major risk factors are high blood pressure, high blood lipid levels and cigarette smoking; and an additional risk factor becoming more apparent, obesity. There is some agreement that diet plays a role in heart disease risk, but it may well be the amount of calories in and calories out more than whether or not these calories come from animal or vegetable fats. Whether or not obesity is an independent risk factor is a scientific question; however, on a public policy basis it is a risk factor dominant in most populations due to its association with hyperlipidemia, hypertension, glucose intolerance and sedentary lifestyles. It would seem that the attainment of ideal body weights in the population would go far in reducing heart disease risk. Much is made of the implementation of the dietary intervention approach to risk reduction as compared to weight reduction, possibly because it is easier to change everyone's diet than it is to change an individual's body weight.

Is a health policy directed at reducing the prevalence of obesity feasible? Possibly as much so as a policy to change the overall diet! There are really only two ways to maintain an ideal body weight in the patient prone to gain weight – reduce caloric intake or increase caloric output. We hear and read a great deal about the benefits of exercise, which is certainly justified, yet there are few if any attempts to raise the next generation of adults with the habits of regular exercise and proper dietary habits. The epidemiologists often point to the Japanese lifestyle as one suitable for a low incidence of heart disease; however, there are more differences than dietary fat and cholesterol intakes which separate our two cultures and could conceivably account for differences in heart disease incidence. One striking difference is the more pronounced emphasis on organized sports in the Japanese society, including the workplace. A leaner, trimmer, fitter society could well be the health policy needed to attack the epidemic of heart disease we currently experience. Some evidence for the benefits of such a life-style has been demonstrated in studies of farmers and urban dwellers which have shown that farmers have lower heart disease mortality rates even though they consume more total calories, cholesterol and animal fat and have slightly higher plasma cholesterol levels. Two consistent differences between urban and rural populations are smoking habits and overall fitness and vigorous exercise.

9 Change diets but not according to the faddist extremists

Mankind now experiences the longest life expectancy ever known; in many ways due to advances in medicine and to better overall nutrition, both quality and quantity. It seems curious that the diet we now enjoy, which has in part provided this extension of the lifespan, is accused of being the culprit in the development of a number of diseases associated with ageing. Should the population change its diet to reduce the risks of these degenerative diseases? Yes, but not necessarily to the patterns being proposed by some organisations. Moderation, a variety of foods, the recommended daily requirements of vitamins and minerals and caloric restriction to attain and maintain ideal body weight are changes well worth incorporating into the public's eating habits. Efforts to educate the public regarding the value of high quality nutrients and the wasted food dollar spent on empty calorie 'junk foods' would seem to make better health sense than the scare tactics required to develop a 'good food, bad food' mentality towards some very valuable dietary constituents.

Nutrition is a science challenged by the same rigours of evidence as any other scientific discipline. Unfortunately nutrition is also a catch phrase used by many with little or no nutritional science training. Today's snake oil salesmen now write popular books on nutrition and play on man's fear of mortality by promising much more than is reasonable let alone proven. Yet the public's fascination with diet and health is understandable and as long as the scientific community argues the pros and cons of mass dietary changes (a valuable part of the scientific process asking questions and demanding answers), the way will be clear for those promising eternal health and vigour by eating their prescribed diet. The clinical-scientist is frustrated by the need to do something to alleviate this epidemic of heart disease while striving to document the proof of benefit and lack of harm of whatever dietary intervention is proposed. We cannot be sure at this stage of our understanding of the causes and treatment of heart disease that any recommended diet is effective in reducing risk when applied to the general public. That is not to say that dietary interventions are not recommended for the hypercholesterolemic patient, yet even here one cannot be assured that dietary treatment of elevated blood cholesterol levels, even when effective, will significantly reduce heart disease risk.

10 Recommendations: for individuals not populations

The outcome of much of this scientific debate with its public exposure and the pronouncements from pseudo-nutritionists is a confused and cynical public. What should an individual do to reduce his or her risk of heart disease? First find out which risk factors exist and which ones can be reduced by some type of intervention. Reasonable suggestions but so often not paid attention to. Is the plasma cholesterol level elevated and if so, what specific dietary changes effectively lower it? Is the individual overweight, hypertensive, a chain smoker, sedentary and mildly diabetic? What life-style changes can be made to reduce overall heart disease risk? These are basic questions which require more of the patient than to give up eating eggs, red meats, and dairy products; however, they also have the potential of making significant changes in that patient's heart disease risk profile. And of even greater potential benefit is that this approach treats those who need treatment in an effective, patient-specific manner and allows the rest of us to feel less guilty and apprehensive about what we are having for dinner tonight.

Notes and References

H.C. McGill, 'The relationship of dietary cholesterol to serum cholesterol concentration and to atherosclerosis in man' in *American Journal of Clinical Nutrition*, Vol. 32, 1979, pp.2664–2702.

Food and Nutrition Board, National Research Council, *Guidelines Toward Healthful Diets*, National Academy of Science, Washington DC, 1980.

S.M. Grundy, D. Bilheimer, H. Blackburn, W.V. Brown, P.O. Kwiterovich Jr., F. Mattson, G. Schonfeld, W.H. Weidman, *Rationale of the diet-heart statement of the American Heart Association*, Circulation Vol. 65, 1985, 839–854A.

E.H. Ahrens Jr., 'Dietary fat and coronary heart disease: unfinished business' in *Lancet*, Vol. 2, 1982, pp. 1121–1124.

D.J. McNamara, 'Diet and hyperlipidemia: a justifiable debate', *Archive of Internal-Medicine*, Vol. 142, 1982, pp. 1345–1348.

P. Samuel, D.J. McNamara, J. Shapiro, 'The role of diet in the etiology and treatment of atherosclerosis', *Annual Review of Medicine*, Vol. 34, 1983, pp. 179–194.

4 Salt and High Blood Pressure: A Study in Education, Persuasion and Naivete.

J.D. Swales

1 Pressure from the media on medical researchers is always for a positive message

Once they enter the harsh world of popular communication medical scientists like myself experience a feeling of extraordinary vulnerability. This is more so when clinical researchers as opposed to basic scientists are questioned by the media. If you have discovered a new fact about the outer universe or the genetic constitution of the fruit fly then you are under no obligation to communicate it to the man on the Clapham Omnibus. Wide publicity in this case is likely to be the result of a conscious decision on your part and therefore to serve some particular purpose such as encouraging financial support to come forward or, quite simply, fame. Popular interest (or at least curiosity) may be served, but otherwise people's lives are not directly influenced by the spread of such knowledge. If your research is medical however, you may still be helping to satisfy an insatiable human need for knowledge, but you may also be telling your audience something of immediate relevance to the way in which they live their lives. The two needs can rarely be separated: once you tell people what you have found out it is difficult to prevent yourself telling them what should be done about it. Such advice may be premature, but if there is some simple harmless recommendation, even if it is later proved to be unjustified, by definition surely no-one will be worse off....? And then the tempter murmurs again. A few practical suggestions of course emphasise the relevance of your findings to everyday life. It would show you to be no ivory tower scientist but a genuinely practical, involved man. After all there can be no harm in it.

These are no abstract ruminations. Four years ago Mr. Geoff Watts of the BBC's 'Medicine Now' programme rang up. Some Belgian workers had discovered a relationship between calcium and blood pressure in recruits to the Belgian Army. The higher blood or urine calcium was found to be, the higher the blood pressure in a fairly weak sort of way. Blood pressure research is littered with such associations. There is a simple reason for this. Blood pressure is influenced by a multitude of factors in the environment as well as by the genes you inherit. The level of pressure varies from second to second in response to environmental factors to meet the needs of body tissues for an adequate supply of blood. More long-term influences like external temperature, weight, diet, general health, temperament and level of activity also come into the picture. If all these influences on blood pressure were independent of each other the task would be relatively easy. The trouble is that these factors are not independent. Your blood pressure can reflect not only diet but also the state of your health, your temperament, your level of activity and your social class. It may also reflect the medical advice about diet and lifestyle which you have been given, perhaps as a result of discovering that you have high blood pressure. Even diet is not as simple as it appears at first sight. If you take a lot of calcium in your diet this probably results from a high intake of dairy products which will therefore be correlated with a high intake of animal fat. It will also probably reflect your own beliefs about milk, cheese and 'healthy' foods which may in turn reflect such other less easily defined factors as education and social class. Any of these may either directly or indirectly influence blood pressure. To pick out one factor and identify it as a 'cause' of high blood pressure is therefore hazardous in the extreme.

I explained this to Mr. Watts as best I could, using the usual formula which people tend to favour on these occasions. 'Interesting findings ... requiring confirmation and further studies to interpret their meaning etc....' It was not a particularly exciting or newsworthy message and I suspect that Mr. Watts was a trifle disappointed. Nevertheless he soldiered on 'Did I think it was a wise precaution to advise people who had a high intake of calcium to reduce it as there was a possibility that this might reduce blood pressure?' This at first sight seemed a modest proposal. Indeed seemingly healthy individuals show a wide range of calcium intakes: some consume a lot, some a little without obviously coming to grief. If those who take a lot reduce their dietary calcium to the population average, where would be the harm in that: if there was a causal relationship between blood pressure and calcium they could only benefit? My first feelings about such potential advice were of the 'a plague on all your houses' variety. I have heard dietitians and nutritionists advising reducing sodium, increasing potassium, magnesium, unsaturated fats and dietary fibre as a means of reducing blood pressure.

I would prefer doctors and those who have recently become known as 'health care professionals' to be a little more sure of their ground before sharing their dubious speculative beliefs with the world at large. My actual reply was a marginally dishonest one. I often see patients, I explained to Mr. Watts, whose ill-health was due to the fact that their diet was grossly deficient in calcium and it would seem foolish to submit otherwise healthy people to such a risk. The facts were true, but of course Mr. Watts was not arguing in favour of the strict vegetarian diet which produces problems of calcium deficiency and bone disease: a modest reduction in dairy product intake would not have such disastrous effects. Nevertheless, Mr. Watts does not subject his guests to hostile interrogation and I was allowed to wriggle off the hook by my intellectual sleight of hand. Which is just as well. Four years later McCarron was demonstrating a *negative* association between dietary calcium and blood pressure and concluding that a *high* intake of dairy products and calcium protected against high blood pressure. I then found myself consulted by the Press for a second time. Again I had to put forward an unwelcome conservative view: on this occasion that we should not all be shifting our diet in the opposite direction.

2 Harm from misleading public health nutritional advice is very difficult to demonstrate

I cite this example because it is so easy to succumb to temptation and give the newsworthy reply rather than the cautious, uninspiring alternative. 'After all it can do no harm', is the argument that the devil puts on such occasions. But is this the case? To pursue my example, it is still possible (although improbable in my opinion) that one or other of the calcium hypotheses is correct. If so, then just as much harm (in the form of increased blood pressure) will presumably be caused by adopting a strategy based upon the wrong hypothesis as good will ensue from following the correct advice. If the benefits are considered worthwhile with one policy then harm must be equally undesirable with the opposite. It is an unfortunate fact of public life that those who are responsible for erroneous advice in this context are mercifully unlikely to suffer personally for it. The consequences of a population change of blood pressure will be spread over many years, the advisers will be long forgotten if the consequences of their erroneous advice are in fact ever analysed. Even that analysis is extraordinarily difficult because of the certainty that many other factors which influence blood pressure will be altering simultaneously. The task of sorting it out may well be beyond our successors.

The calcium hypothesis is a newcomer to the field, although it too has attracted its evangelists. The salt hypothesis is much older. Although there was evidence dating back to the turn of the century that reducing salt intake lowered blood pressure in certain patients, the hypothesis that salt was a cause of hypertension (high blood pressure) in man was only formally enunciated by Dahl thirty years ago. In brief, Dahl's hypothesis was based upon two lines of reasoning. Firstly he claimed there was a direct relationship between the incidence of hypertension and the use of salt in a variety of societies across the world. Secondly, he bred a strain of rat which became hypertensive when a large amount of sodium was given with its food: this strain of rat continued to have a high blood pressure even when salt was reduced. This predisposition to high blood pressure seemed to be related to some change in kidney function since hypertension could be transferred by kidney transplantation.

3 The popularity of the salt hypothesis occurred in response to a need rather than an accumulation of scientific evidence

Dahl's hypothesis was not generally accepted at the time. The anthropological data on which it was based were too uncertain and the Dahl strain of rat did not seem to have many similarities with other forms of hypertension in laboratory animals. Enthusiasm for the hypothesis only developed in the late 1970s. The reason for this is itself revealing. Little fresh evidence was available but the medical climate had changed. The importance of hypertension as a treatable risk factor in cardiovascular disease became recognised. Cardiovascular disease is the major health problem of Western society. The need to treat more and more otherwise healthy individuals with high blood pressure became frightening. The cost and the organisational problems posed by a life-time's drug treatment of up to 20 per cent of the adult population were seen as an appalling challenge. How much nicer if a simple change in habit could have the same effect. By lowering blood pressure at an earlier stage it might even be more effective than drug treatment. How even more congenial if that change took the form of rooting out one of the dietary aberrations of modern industrial civilisation which had given rise to the disorder in the first place. Perhaps after all Dahl was right and there was a lesson we could all learn from the Rousseau-like innocence of primitive peoples who had no hypertension and ate little salt, or perhaps we should take as an example the Dahl strain of rat before the experimentator laced its diet generously with this toxic substance. The concept was simple, it gripped the imagination and was easily communicated.

The mission started in America but soon spread to certain parts of the continent of Europe. Finally our own Health Education Council entered the field with a series of full page advertisements in the tabloids asking us rhetorically 'What Shook 100 Million Americans into Eating Less Salt.' Underneath we were told 'Doctors suggest that we are eating too much'. We are then told about the worldwide studies on eating salt and blood pressure. The claim is not made, and in my experience never is, that the matter is proven up to the hilt. On the other hand these advertisements imply again, where is the harm in it? There is of course a flaw in the logic here as I have indicated and I will later document the potential harm which has to be set against the equally potential good. There is another equally obvious concern. Because our belief is highly convenient at a particular point in history this can scarcely be regarded as validating that belief. We do not have to look far for an example of what happens when political pressure influences scientific research. Lysenko's studies of the influence of environmental factors upon genetic determinants were congenial to the political theory of his masters and his work prospered for a while as a result. However, the long-term effect was disastrous for Soviet science. We have therefore to distinguish between an idea that has found its time and an idea that owes its acceptance to a current need.

4 Two semi-official reports give a spurious sense of respectability to the salt hypothesis

There is no doubt that the prevention of high blood pressure or even a slight reduction in blood pressure in the population carries the prospect of enormous benefit. Because it is so important and because it is probably achievable it seems to me critically important that we get it right. Let us therefore look in a little more detail at the case for a reduction in population salt intake. Two widely cited reports have made this proposal. Most admit that the evidence is by no means conclusive: both were more concerned with lipid and fibre intake and neither showed evidence of particular familiarity with blood pressure research. However, they are usually quoted as authoritative pronouncements.

The Committee on Medical Aspects of Food Policy (COMA) was set up by the DHSS. Its findings on salt were tentatively expressed: 'The Panel recommends that the dietary intake of common salt should not be increased further and that consideration should be given to ways and means of decreasing it.' Since the first proposition is not seriously maintained by anyone, the second is the only relevant suggestion. It is supported by a further statement that 'We believe that the intake of salt in the United Kingdom diet (approximately 7–10 grams per day) is needlessly high'. For evidence we are referred to another section of the report which refers to the cross-cultural studies again which 'show a statistical association between estimates of salt intake and average blood pressure'. The report goes on to weaken the value of this evidence by referring to the possible effects of 'weight gain, high fat and low potassium intake in promoting a rise in blood pressure' and rather vaguely cites community studies in Finland and Belgium which suggest that 'a variety of dietary changes do lead to a fall in average blood pressure'. Some feeding trials, we are told, have shown that small reductions in blood pressure occur when salt intake is deliberately reduced. We are given no references to such studies other than a World Health Organisation Report.

The National Advisory Committee on Nutrition Education (NACNE) Report was published by the Health Education Council. It concluded that the (average) salt intake of 12 grams a day was 'far in excess of that required even by physically active individuals' and that 'a gradual reduction to half or even a quarter of this level is unlikely to be associated with any danger to health'. Since there was no data on possible harm the latter statement has a quality of hope about it rather than conviction. Nevertheless the NACNE Report does offer citation to the scientific literature and on these grounds enables us to assess the quality of supporting evidence.

5 The Dahl 'salt sensitive' rat is irrelevant to the problem

'Experiments in animals' we are told 'have shown that very high intakes of sodium lead to high levels of blood pressure and that modest intakes of sodium (although still above that naturally occurring in the animals' food) can lead to hypertension in genetically susceptible animals'. The reference cited to this is to a paper published in 1962 by Louis Dahl the originator of the salt hypothesis.

The Dahl rat has a slightly bewildering quality of appearing and disappearing like the Cheshire Cat in discussions on salt. It is often cited confidently, frequently with the misleading implication that the features which it manifests are common to all strains of rat. When the literature of experimental hypertension is examined more critically it usually vanishes from the discussion and we are told that animal experimentation is irrelevant. This ignores the fact that Dahl's original hypothesis depended substantially on such experimentation.

The first and most telling point about the Dahl rat perhaps centres on the description of the salt intake needed to produce hypertension as 'modest'. In the paper quoted, eight grams of salt per 100 grams of food were used. This is equivalent to twenty times the normal salt intake of a rat and if extrapolated to a healthy man would produce dramatic circulatory consequences. This level of salt intake would however soon become quite intolerable. The use of a publication dating back to 1962 is itself perhaps worthy of comment. This is an early study on the metabolism of sodium and hypertension: a vast amount of work has been carried out in the succeeding two decades. Certainly the Dahl paper is often cited in scientific reviews but now usually in a historical context only. It is also interesting to note that however persuasive the paper was to NACNE, it did not persuade the scientific community at the time of the truth of the Dahl hypothesis. But why not quote more recent papers on the Dahl rat? There has been a profusion of such papers. Perhaps the NACNE writers did not appreciate that Dahl later changed his view of the unique sensitivity of his strain to salt. In one of his last papers in 1974 he ceases to refer to 'salt sensitivity' at all. To quote that paper (which now refers to a 'sensitive' rather than 'salt-sensitive' strain). 'Separation of strains was originally based on sharply different blood pressure responses to a high sodium intake. It was found subsequently that the disparate blood pressure responses were not unique to a sodium stimulus but rather indicative of separate opposite reactions to hypertensinogenic stimuli generally'. In other words the Dahl sensitive rat is a rat in which blood pressure is very susceptible to stress. If scientific balance is to be achieved it is perhaps relevant to mention other ways of inducing high blood pressure. In one of the most commonly used laboratory strains of rat severe salt *restriction* raises blood pressure as it does in rats with hypertension caused by disease of one kidney. To produce this sort of response salt intake has to be reduced to less than 10 per cent and it seems likely that this too is due to the effect of the stress of an abnormal diet: clearly one would not like to place too much importance on either phenomenon. It simply underlines the fact that everything is not as simple as it seems when one adopts a very selective approach to an extremely complex literature.

6 Cross-cultural studies show that environmental factors are important, nothing more

The NACNE Report pays most attention to the cross-cultural studies, citing such hypertension-free societies as the Yanamamo Indians, the Bushmen and the Samburu Warriors. The Report goes on to cite a review by Lilian Glieberman of 27 populations across the world in which there was a 'linear relation of both systolic and diastolic blood pressures and salt intake'. Glieberman's paper published in 1973 has the merit of citing the source of her evidence. Dahl's paper did not make this clear. Glieberman reviews retrospectively a variety of papers published in the medical and anthropological literature over the previous two decades. In most cases the authors were not primarily looking at blood pressure and salt intake. In 10 of the cited studies there was no indication of how salt intake was measured and in six Glieberman estimated what the salt intake could have been from dietary descriptions. Dietary histories are notoriously unreliable and in the circumstances in which they were carried out the problems must have been formidable, bearing in mind the contradictions in the COMA and NACNE reports when they considered average salt intake in our relatively well-documented culture. Glieberman was only concerned with the possible role of sodium. Other factors were not measured. The NACNE Report is clearly uneasy about this: elsewhere they mention other dietary factors which may possibly have played a role in hypertension-free societies such as 'lack of obesity, high levels of physical activity, low animal fat diets and a high dietary intake of potassium'. Since Glieberman did not look at these factors their importance is impossible to assess. It is notable that she does not attach the same weight to her findings which others have subsequently done and concludes that to assess the possible role of salt in blood pressure 'more refined, in depth analyses are required'. Since her review, careful scientific studies have shown that adopting a vegetarian diet or restricting fat intake (together perhaps with an increase in unsaturated fat) lowers blood pressure significantly without altering salt intake. The low-salt cultures are high in vegetable matter and low in animal fat. Were appropriate crosscultural data available the association between blood pressure and animal fats could well be as good as that between salt and blood pressure. It might prove to be better. Unfortunately the studies are too sketchy for this type of analysis to be carried out.

Other factors may also be relevant. One of the most widely hypertension-free groups to be investigated has been the rural black African. By contrast hypertension assumes Western proportions when the black migrates to the city. Whilst his diet clearly alters, many other relevant influences also alter. In an extensive series of studies in Durban, Y.K. Seedat found that higher blood pressure levels in the black were associated with a higher incidence of insomnia due to anxiety, cigarette smoking, alcohol, poorer conditions of work, lower educational status, greater number of children not working, lack of recreation and overcrowding in homes. The difficulty is that food in urban societies tends to be high in sodium: when blood pressure rises as individuals migrate to such societies it is not therefore surprising that assumption of a high salt diet and a rise in blood pressure go together: other things are also altering simultaneously. It is certainly not justifiable to conclude that when two factors alter in parallel they are cause and effect.

Finally it is apparent from the graph which Glieberman draws that the relationship between salt intake and blood pressure is largely dependent upon five sets of observations representing low blood pressures in cultures apparently consuming less than four grams of salt per day. Above this level the relationship is unconvincing. The proposal put forward by NACNE is for an annual reduction in intake of one gram of salt per day for five years which would still leave salt intake well above this level. Assuming the validity of the Glieberman study those who apply it have to assume a straight-line relationship between salt intake and blood pressure so that a modest reduction in salt intake produces a modest reduction in blood pressure. This relationship is certainly not evident from the data which Glieberman presents. The NACNE Report does not tell us why they selected the magic figure of five grams of salt a day rather than a reduction of eight grams or two grams. This is not perhaps surprising as there have been no long-term studies on the effects of different levels of salt intake in the same group of individuals.

The low-salt cultures always figure most prominently in the writings of the advocates of salt restriction and in their advertising propaganda. The reason is fairly clear: more direct evidence is not available. Nevertheless the principle is a surprising one which should not be allowed to pass unquestioned. It would be quite unique in medicine for the lifestyle of primitive (and relatively short-lived) peoples to serve as a model for health practices of Western populations.

7 Patients with high blood pressure do not eat more salt than healthy individuals

The NACNE Report admits that within cultural studies have failed to show that hypertensive patients have a higher intake of salt than the rest of the population. This had indeed been a quite consistent observation which sets salt intake and blood pressure in a separate category from say blood cholesterol and coronary heart disease. It is also worth pointing out that epidemiological studies have had no difficulty in demonstrating a consistent relationship between obesity or alcohol and blood pressure. Several studies for instance have convincingly shown that vegetarians *within a single population* have lower blood pressures at all ages than omnivores. The failure to demonstrate a relationship between salt intake and blood pressure is therefore at first sight disconcerting. The explanation given is that individuals are likely to vary in their genetic susceptibility to salt-induced hypertension 'so a failure to distinguish between susceptible and non-susceptible individuals may explain the poor relationship between salt intake and blood pressure within a population.' This explanation should be seen for what it is: a retrospective hypothesis to explain an uncongenial but generally agreed observation. A Finnish group claimed that relatives of hypertensive patients did show a relationship between sodium intake and blood pressure. This brief report (which is cited in the NACNE document) was subsequently criticised for fundamental faults in design since it ignored the role of differences in body weight as causes of differences in blood pressure: it has not been reproduced by a more careful study from Glasgow. There are good theoretical reasons for believing that the population cannot be divided into salt susceptible and non-salt susceptible individuals unless these effects are in some way graded. The genetic susceptibility hypothesis has the aroma of special pleading about it.

8 There is no evidence that restricting salt intake lowers blood pressure in healthy individuals

If adequate scientific investigation is impossibly difficult it could be argued that action is necessary on the balance of probability. This is the point at which my perplexity evolves into frank astonishment. When we discuss possible ways of reducing say deaths from coronary heart disease we need very large studies of large numbers of people followed for many years, simply because relatively few individuals will suffer a heart attack in the period of study and we have to show a reduction in that number. This difficulty exists because we cannot easily measure or follow changes in the severity of coronary artery disease. Blood pressure measurement is outstandingly simple and pain-free. If we are carrying out a manoeuvre which is claimed to change blood pressure this can be quite simply put to the test. Why one might ask should we bother at all with the primitive peoples if this is the case? The NACNE Report wisely does not use the argument which is occasionally put forward by some of the more enthusiastic if uncritical advocates of salt restriction i.e. that the effect of salt is only apparent after years of exposure. There is nothing in our knowledge of the physiological systems which maintain blood pressure to suggest that salt would have such a 'slow' effect. Further when other dietary influences on blood pressure are examined (such as alcohol, vegetarian diet, dietary lipids) significant effects of dietary change on blood pressure can be demonstrated within a week or two.

9 What is the result of restricting salt intake therefore?

To quote the NACNE Report 'Metabolic experiments in human beings have demonstrated a fall in blood pressure when subjects are fed a low sodium diet'. Three papers are cited in favour of this contention. Two of these are misquoted in this context since they deal not with the healthy population, but with patients selected because they have established high blood pressure. The NACNE Report does not point this out, and the implication therefore is grossly misleading. The third study deals with healthy subjects with normal blood pressure but, despite the assertion of the NACNE Report to the contrary, was able to find no significant change in blood pressure with salt restriction. Not mentioned by NACNE is the fact that salt restriction and loading of a non-extreme degree has consistently failed to influence blood pressure in a series of studies carried out in North America, the United Kingdom and Europe. Two studies which recorded a positive result have little relevance to the current discussion. In one blood pressure rose by a small extent when salt intake was increased tenfold. The other study showed a very small increase in systolic blood pressure when sodium intake in newborn infants was raised threefold for the first six months of life. Blood pressure then fell to normal. The authors of that report later carried out a study of salt restriction in adults with borderline hypertension and could demonstrate no influence upon blood pressure.

The effect of salt restriction upon high blood pressure levels is more controversial. Some studies have shown a small but significant fall in blood pressure: other studies have not. These reports are not as inconsistent as they appear at first sight. Salt restriction seems to have little effect on the milder degrees of high blood pressure. Some patients with more severe hypertension do seem to show some effect of salt restriction. This is particularly the case if they are already receiving some forms of blood pressure lowering drugs. Salt restriction may therefore be helpful in some cases to a minor degree although it alone is usually insufficient to bring blood pressure down to normal. For the remaining patients and for the rest of the population it seems to have little effect. Even when blood pressure is lowered this tells us nothing about why it is raised in the first place. Bleeding is an equally effective method of lowering blood pressure yet no-one claims that an excess of blood is responsible. Hypertensive patients have impairment of some of the systems which keep blood pressure constant in the face of changes in body fluids. Without the protection offered by these usually extremely effective systems the loss of body fluids produced by salt restriction would produce an effect which it would not do under normal circumstances. The salt 'sensitivity' of some hypertensive patients therefore appears to be a consequence and not a cause of high blood pressure.

10 There is no evidence that a hypertensive patient's body contains too much salt

Despite a predilection for the Dahl rat, health educationists' propaganda does not usually mention the most obvious physiological characteristic of the hypertensive man. The NACNE Report is not alone in keeping silent on this point. When as a result of disease or certain medications, body salt content is increased the immediate consequence is retention of water as well. This extra water is observed in the blood (plasma) and in the fluids contained in body tissues. In high blood pressure, plasma volume is *reduced* in proportion to the degree of blood pressure elevation: the higher the blood pressure in general the smaller the plasma volume. Further, three studies have reported that the early stages of high blood pressure are associated with a *decrease* in body sodium content. Although the literature now includes more than 20 reports of measurement of body sodium using radioactive isotopes, to the best of my knowledge not one scientifically-respectable study has managed to demonstrate an increase in body sodium in patients with high blood pressure provided we exclude certain rare diseases which cause high blood pressure. It has occasionally been argued that there may be too much sodium in certain parts of the circulation which is not demonstrated by these methods, but such arguments remain unconvincing in their special pleading. Equally, and perhaps more surprisingly, even the Dahl salt-sensitive rat consuming its massive quantities of salt shows no evidence of an increase in body sodium.

11 The literature of high blood pressure research is so extensive that selective citations can produce any conclusion

But surely even if each item of evidence alone is not particularly persuasive the sum total of evidence is suggestive? The sceptic is always at a disadvantage when on the defensive. Even if his doubts are justified in some cases is it not probable that one piece of evidence does contain some nugget of truth? Perhaps the sceptics do protest too much. Not many scientists would share such a view but it clearly has its attractions. It is however an extremely dangerous argument. The fallacy lies in the volume of scientific literature on high blood pressure and the opportunity which this conveys for selective citation.

Six times a year the American Heart Association publishes a recurring bibliography of hypertension in which papers published in the more reputable scientific journals are listed. Each two-month bibliography contains 2,000–3,000 references (allowing for some repetition). Although some of these papers are subject to some sort of peer review before publication the scientific standard of published work is, to say the least, variable. Regrettably in some cases the reputation of the individuals reporting it will give some idea of its value. When a new hypothesis is produced the columns of the bibliography over the next few years are flooded with papers both in favour and against. After a time the dust settles, most of the work is soon forgotten and science moves on. Given an enormous quantity of published data careful selection can readily build up a convincing case. The NACNE Report contains one example of culling the literature for support which is unfortunately a glaring one. The central question in giving population advice is surely: can we reduce blood pressure by such advice? We have seen that small short-term studies would suggest that we could not do this in healthy individuals. On the other hand in the NACNE Report we read 'There are few documented intervention studies but Farquar was able to demonstrate a five mm reduction in mean systolic blood pressure by a modest reduction in salt intake in a sample of the population.' The difficulty with such studies is that most nutritionists (particularly in the United States) prefer to give broad-based advice which changes several components of the diet at the same time: it is particularly likely that dietary fat is reduced at the same time as salt. It is important to examine such studies carefully. On referral to the list of references at the end of the NACNE Report we find that the Farquar study is reported not in a scientific journal or indeed in a scientific paper at all but in the 'Abstracts of the 18th Annual Conference on Cardiovascular Disease Epidemiology, 1978 in the CVD Newsletter no. 28'. Such a citation would not even get into the bibliography of hypertension. The use of such a publication to support a major recommendation is not acceptable scientific practice. When one recalls that it is the only study cited which actually purports to assess the consequences of carrying out a manoeuvre being recommended for the whole population for five years it is fairly apparent that an enormous superstructure is being built on an extremely weak foundation.

12 Selective citations from the literature can prove almost anything

Let me illustrate the misuse of selective citations of the literature in another way. I will put forward another hypothesis and population advice based on it. This could be described as the new anti-Dahl theory. It regards high blood pressure as a disease of inadequate salt intake. As a result we have the reduced plasma volume and evidence of reduced body sodium in the early stages of hypertension in man. In some models in the rat increased blood pressure is associated with sodium loss. In both rats and human patients with very severe hypertension salt has been administered and has improved patients' condition remarkably. By contrast, salt depletion in rats and in one or two studies in man has caused *increased* blood pressure. Cross-cultural studies support the hypothesis really since hypertension has been eliminated from populations with a low salt intake indicating that a combination of the two is disadvantageous and therefore has eliminated the gene responsible for high blood pressure. As a result the population should be encouraged to increase salt intake. I can cite several references in support of each of the above statements: these are full papers by reputable scientific workers. The hypothesis is nevertheless nonsense because it is an unequally one-sided and selective view of the literature as the NACNE Report.

13 There has been no assessment of the possible adverse effects of salt restriction

The NACNE Report states that 'a gradual reduction of salt intake to a half or a quarter is unlikely to be associated with any danger to health'. This may or may not be true. As the consequences of a population reduction in salt intake have not been examined, it is impossible to judge. However, severe salt restriction (i.e. to 10 per cent or less) in animals is associated with a reduced capacity to survive surgery and haemorrhage. Also in animals (and probably in man) it predisposes to acute renal failure and circulatory collapse. It is unlikely that any individual who has reduced his salt intake by say half, will be subject to these medical disasters. What is quite unknown is whether the adverse effects of salt restriction are confined to the extremes or whether they are linearly related to the reduction in salt intake i.e. an adverse effect becomes progressively more likely the further below the population mean we restrict our salt intake. The advocates of a population reduction in salt intake are therefore in the unenviable position of having to argue that the relationship between salt intake and blood pressure is linear (without any evidence to favour this view) whilst maintaining that the relationship between the incidence of adverse effects and salt intake is non-linear and confined to severe salt restriction. There is no evidence to help us reach a conclusion about either and it is therefore impossible to construct a realistic cost-benefit equation.

One other argument is sometimes used in this context as a way of escape from the dilemma. Even if we reduce salt intake very severely, the kidneys reduce their output of salt: if we increase salt intake the excess is put out in the urine. It is concluded that the requirement for salt is very low and that the greater part of our salt intake is needlessly excessive since it is excreted by the kidneys. If this were true, in the literal sense it is difficult to see what harm could result. However, this argument is based on a serious misunderstanding of salt metabolism. Changing salt intake results in an adjustment of a wide range of bodily functions, with alterations in body fluids, blood flow to body tissues and the hormones and nervous system activity which controls the circulation. It is not reasonable to talk of a requirement in this situation without knowing what the optimal state of each of these systems is. We have no idea of this in man until we have studied the effect of sustained alterations in salt intake on a variety of measures of well-being and health. We return therefore to the starting point: we do not have the relevant information on which to form an opinion.

14 Campaigns to reform diet have been started with insufficient consideration of the risk benefit ratio

Why, therefore, are campaigns being mounted if we do not have the necessary evidence: since the evidence is obtainable in a relatively short period of time why is energy and money being put into persuasion rather than into carefully-designed investigation? One cannot escape the conclusion that the wish for a thing to be true has given rise to the belief that it is true. One also has to admit that some reputable scientists (mainly in the United States) have lent their support to a policy of reducing salt intake. Their case is no more persuasive than that produced by the NACNE Report, but they have supported widespread attempts at dietary reform.

Campaigns to change the national diet are more prevalent in the United States and it is undoubtedly easier to make a concerted attack on several fronts: the possibility of success is enhanced even if the blunderbuss approach is somewhat unscientific. This would be reasonable if we have assurance that we were not doing harm. However, only a very small risk is required to balance the small potential individual benefit. The recent MRC Trial in Mild Hypertension indicated that treatment reduced the risk of one stroke in 850 patients followed for one year. This is small enough but the risk and therefore the potential benefit is several-fold less in a healthy population with a normal blood pressure. Are we convinced that reducing salt intake will not also reduce one individual's ability to resist major haemorrhage, surgical operation or gastroenteritis amongst say 2,000 individuals who have also reduced their salt intake in the hope that it may reduce blood pressure? Such adverse effects may occur, no-one knows how frequently.

15 The credentials of the 'dietary expert' should be looked at carefully

The 'majority of experts', Which Magazine informed its readers, felt that dietary salt should be reduced. These issues were also rehearsed vigorously in the columns of the *Lancet* in 1984. Several of us put forward the case for caution until reasonable scientific evidence gave us better guidance emphasising that this was an instance where information could be obtained within a reasonable period. The signatories of the letter included the President, Past-President and Vice-President of the British Hypertension Society (the learned Society for high blood pressure research in the United Kingdom), The President of the International Society of Hypertension and senior members of the Medical Research Council Blood Pressure Unit (the largest research group working in this area in the United Kingdom), and the Professor of Cardiology at Cornell University who is one of the best known international workers in this area. The first reply came from Professor Alwyn Smith who put forward the case for a reduction in salt intake. Amongst other things he makes one revealing statement. 'That [present salt intake] may contribute to prevalent blood pressure levels and therefore to cerebrovascular and coronary artery disease mortality is as widely agreed as any proposition in medicine is likely to be'. The media who took up the controversy presented the two letters as illustrating experts in disarray. A more relevant question could be put. Who are the experts? I happen to know and respect Professor Alwyn Smith who is President of the Faculty of Community Medicine of the Royal College of Physicians. His comments on the problems of the health service and the organisation of medical care are perceptive and valuable. He is not, and I am sure he would not claim to be, an authority on high blood pressure and as far as I know has never published a single paper on the subject. What scientific studies led him to his conclusion are not made clear in his letter. His expertise lies in applying scientific advice to health measures in the community. If we felt salt intake should be reduced he would clearly be the man to approach. Unfortunately we have not yet reached this stage. Apart from Professor Alwyn Smith we have two other sorts of experts on a healthy diet who were doubtless consulted by the Consumers Association and constitute therefore the 'majority of experts'.

These are the health educators and the nutritionists. At least one university now has a Professor of Health Education and several universities have courses in nutrition. Nutrition is indeed an established health care profession. Who it might be asked should know more about what we should be eating than the latter? Unfortunately the role of the nutritionist is much more restricted than that. Ask the average hospital nutritionist how you should restrict your calorie or salt intake and (usually she) can provide a detailed and instructive diet which achieves this aim complete with recipes and specimen meals. The nutritionist working in a university research establishment will probably be studying the effects of food upon particular body biochemical processes. Neither will be familiar with the expanding literature on high blood pressure. It would be unfair to expect them to be familiar with this literature. Both have an established role but analysing the effect of diet on blood pressure is not part of their brief.

The 'health educator' will also be the person to whom the media turn automatically. He will be an individual with a high public profile. He will not necessarily be scientifically trained; he will be superficially familiar with the literature and this will help him to make his case. He will also want a simple and clear message, for success depends upon this. And what if the message is not simple and clear? This presents him with an ugly dilemma. The temptation will be to simplify and clarify it.

Those who carry out medical research are not on the whole elitist. They feel that the arguments should be put, information examined and conclusions reached. If they find individuals making authoritative statements who have no qualifications to do so, this does not cause undue concern. Prejudice and error will in the end, it is felt, inevitably decline as new and better information becomes available. Why therefore enter a public debate when issues are being simplified and distorted out of recognition? Comment about the qualifications of individuals who pontificate is unnecessary and in rather bad taste since in the end right will triumph. Some of us are now finding this approach a trifle naive.

If a head count of experts in hypertension in the United Kingdom was carried out the majority would be sceptical about the case for population salt restriction. Even those who had given their support for the case accept that it is uncertain but support it because on the whole they feel it is unlikely to do harm. The trouble is that the dietary scene includes a variety of experts with dubious credentials. Some are government-funded through the Health Education Council. Having at some stage accepted the case for salt restriction and having entered the public arena they find it difficult to turn back. The health educationist will be reassured in one respect even if the message changes. To misquote Harold Wilson, a year is a long time in health education. The 'healthy diet' of milk, eggs and cheese of a few years back is now mercifully forgotten. And so, if in a few years' time we are told that a reduced calcium, lipid or animal protein intake is the key to low blood pressure the earlier advice will have been forgotten in the evangelical fervour of the new campaign.

Commercial interests have also been involved although not exclusively on one side. The Salt Manufacturers are balanced by the makers of widely-advertised health foods and the publishers and authors of diet books. The outcome seems to depend on factors quite remote from possible benefit. Should those of us actively involved in the study of this field keep silent? There are some who believe we should. This seems to me to be a form of dishonesty incompatible with our scientific credentials. Should we participate although passively in a conspiracy to present as established fact what many of us believe to be dubious speculation so that people take advice which they might otherwise not be prepared to take if they were in full possession of the facts? It is reasonable that society should protect its members, but protection surely does not extend to pretence and falsification. The salt debate involves issues more wide-ranging than the control of blood pressure and its risks.

Notes and References

References to the original papers on which the above is based will be found in my article, 'Dietary Salt and Hypertension' in *Lancet*, No. i, 1980, pp. 1177–1179; the more recent article from the Glasgow MRC Blood Pressure Unit, J.J. Brown, A.F. Lever, J.I.S. Robertson, P. Semple, 'Should Dietary Salt be Reduced: the Sceptics' Position', *Quarterly Journal of Medicine*, No. 53, 1984, pp. 427–435; and the correspondence in the columns of the *Lancet* which began with publication of the letter from Brown et al., '*Salt and Hypertension*', in *Lancet*, No. ii, 1985, p. 456.

5 Fibre: Too Much Speculation, Not Enough Facts

Ian Macdonald

1 Modern food over-refined?

In 1966 a book was published with the basic theme that the food and particularly the carbohydrate containing food eaten in the Western World was too refined. The implication was that in the process of refining the food some desirable components had been removed and it was the absence of these components that accounted for the increased incidence of some diseases in the Western World, when compared with less industrialised countries. Though the book was thin in cause-and-effect data that were scientifically acceptable, the concept was to give rise to considerable interest and to new thinking about the cause of those diseases thought to be due to nutritional abundance. It was perhaps the first time that serious thought had been given to the possible harmful role of modern food (apart from additives), the main concern less than 50 years earlier being nutritional deprivation. From this book, which must surely be a landmark in nutritional thinking, much of the discussions about fibre in the diet arose.

2 'Little in the way of fact'

The concept that a constituent of the diet that is not absorbed or even metabolized can influence metabolism is a notion alien to those whose interests lie in the study of the biochemistry of health and disease. The 'blotting paper' effect of dietary fibre raises a series of intriguing questions, not only as to how this effect is brought about, but also as to what substances present in the gut are absorbed by this 'blotting paper' and how this absorption and subsequent elimination affect the present and future well-being of the individual. Currently there are very few answers to these and other related questions when applied to man largely because some of the apparently desirable effects claimed for fibre are only highlighted after many years of 'fibre deficiency'. Because there is little in the way of fact, though it is increasing, there is an abundance of speculation on the role of dietary fibre in the prevention of disease, and some of the speculators display a fervour not often seen in science.

The current widespread interest in dietary fibre is not confined to those whose main interest is in medicine and nutrition; the imagination of the lay person has been captured by the belief that fibre is a 'health' food. This attitude is possibly part of the generally held view that modern technology has some side effects that could be undesirable and that maybe modern food in the Western World can be too purified. It is, therefore, important to try to make an assessment of the current situation regarding the role of dietary fibre in health and disease that is based on fact. Since the definition of dietary fibre is unclear as is the method of measurement, it is not possible to state whether or not dietary fibre deficiency – or excess – exists.

3 The evidence of geographic pathology: is the different diet of less-developed countries responsible for their rare occurrence of certain diseases?

In 1970 Burkitt, who spent many years as a surgeon in Africa and whose meticulous observations led to the identification of a new form of cancer in children, put forward the view that 'there is reason to suspect a common or related cause for diseases which are both associated with one another in their geographical distribution and tend to occur together in the same patients'. He pointed out that such diseases as diabetes, obesity, atherosclerosis, and noninfective bowel disease such as diverticulosis, polyps, cancer and ulcerative colitis are consistently rare or absent in rural populations in developing countries and consistently common in all economically developed countries. Burkitt then postulated that the ingestible fibre found in the food of the developing countries, which is removed in the processing of sugar and white flour, was the factor responsible for the rarity of the diseases listed above. This hypothesis was similar to one put forward earlier under the generic name 'the saccharine diseases'. Those diseases are supposedly associated with the consumption of refined carbohydrate either as white flour or as sugar. The efficacy, in an uncontrolled trial of unprocessed bran in the treatment of diverticular disease of the colon was reported in 1972. In this report the author made the following statement 'The trial was not controlled for we believe that fibre deficiency causes diverticulosis and hence it would have been unethical for us to have given a low residue diet'.

Another problem in relating dietary fibre to the prevention or treatment of disease, especially in geographical studies, is that many of the diets eaten in different parts of the world, which appear to differ in the amount of fibre they contain also differ qualitatively in other respects and it is important to consider the possible effects of the other changes before ascribing everything to dietary fibre.

A report in the *Lancet* in 1985 noted that mortality rates from colon cancer in the USA are highest in populations exposed to the least amounts of natural sunlight. The high fibre consumers of Africa are probably exposed to more natural sunlight as well as consuming more fibre and could it be the sunlight and not the fibre that is responsible for the possible reduced incidence of colon cancer in Africa? This may be an example of the failure to consider other variables when drawing conclusions from associations.

The evidence presented by those authors who postulate the virtues of dietary fibre is circumstantial and as such is capable of other interpretations; their evidence is more in the nature of an association than a relationship. It is difficult to obtain reliable figures for the incidence of various diseases in rural areas in developing countries and the assumption that colonic diverticula are rare in the East, where the intake of fibre is high, has been challenged. The high incidence of coronary heart disease and cancer of the intestinal tract is in older age groups and therefore seen in higher proportion in the West owing to the greater longevity and better diagnostic resources found there.

4 The evidence from epidemiology: correlations are not necessarily causes

Much of the case supporting the importance to health of dietary fibre comes from surveys which show, for example, a low incidence of a certain disease in a community having a high intake of fibre. Though this is entirely acceptable statistically it can be misleading. Figure 1 shows that life span in the UK has increased along with the average sugar intake in the UK over the past 200 years, but it would not be sensible to ascribe the increased life expectancy to sugar. Figure 2 shows similar comparisons for the dietary fibre intake and again it would be utterly unreasonable to conclude that increased life expectancy in the UK is due to a reduction in fibre intake even though Figure 3 supports this conclusion.

Perhaps of closer interest is the observation that with an increase in fibre intake there may be an increase in stomach cancer (Figure 4). Using the same technique an increased fibre intake is associated with a reduction in colon cancer (Figure 5). If the latter association is accepted as causal why not the former – in fact do we substitute one ill for another?

It would be prudent before offering any widespread advice, to be aware of any possible dangers arising as a result of this advice.

Figure 1: A positive association in the UK between life expectancy and sugar intake.

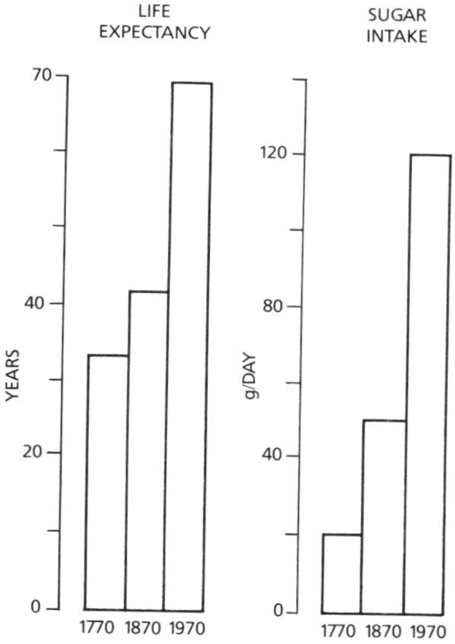

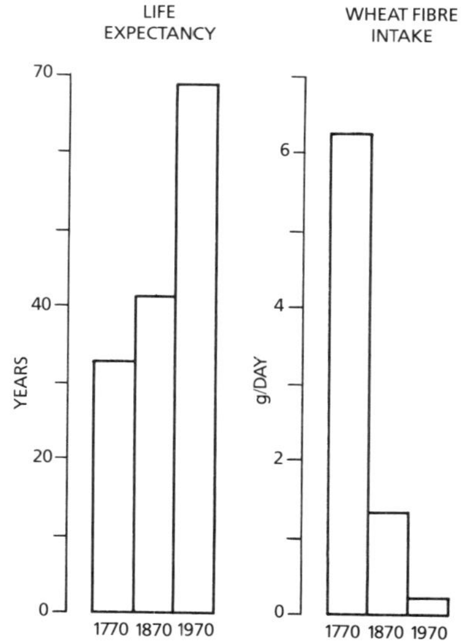

Figure 2: Life expectancy at birth in the UK over two centuries and wheat fibre intake at comparable times showing a negative association of the two parameters.

Figure 3: Showing a negative association in 33 countries between fibre 'intake' and life expectancy. (Data from 10 years of age eliminate the contribution to life expectancy brought by infant mortality. Fibre disappearance is a measure of intake.)

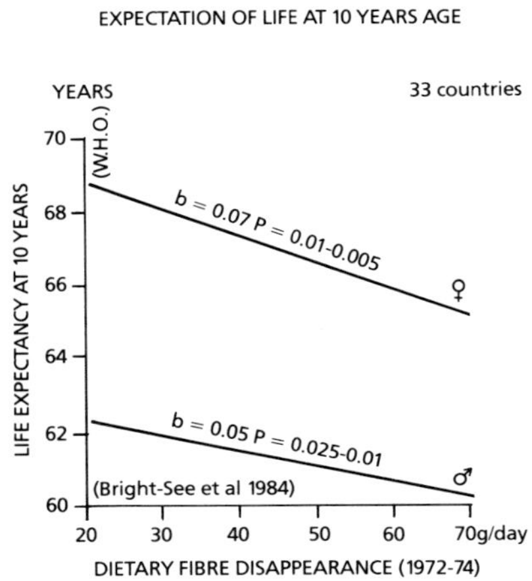

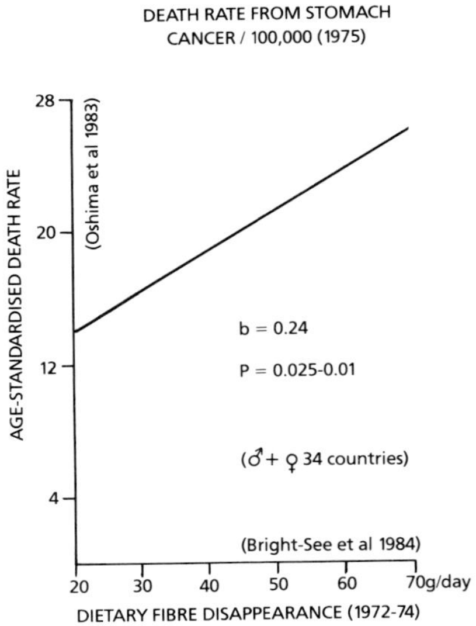

Figure 4: A positive association between dietary fibre 'intake' and death rate from stomach cancer.

Figure 5: A negative association between dietary fibre 'intake' and the incidence/mortality of colo-rectal/colon cancer.

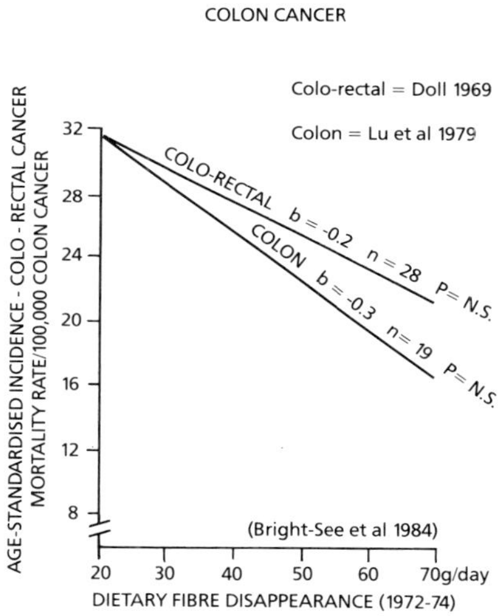

5 The fibre hypothesis should be more modestly and carefully defined in the light of evidence

In any hypothesis, it is not unreasonable to make assumptions, and the use of teleology is acceptable; to persist when the assumptions are either incorrect or of a second or third order weakens the hypothesis. The plateau in the mortality from diverticular disease of the colon in the United Kingdom started in 1933, some six years before the wartime increase in flour extraction. This could be due to the introduction of roller-milled flour in 1880, 50 or so years earlier. However, in the mid-1950s the mortality from diverticular disease in women started to rise and currently is about twice that of men. This sudden appearance of great susceptibility in the female cannot be attributed to changes in milling in 1880–1890.

A decrease in intestinal transit time when fibre is added to the diet has been assumed to be advantageous in itself and from this a second-order assumption is made that slow transit not only allows potential carcinogens to be formed by colonic organisms but also allows increased contact time of the carcinogens with the mucosa of the colon. However, doubt has been thrown on whether fibre does, in fact, decrease transit time in most people.

It has been stated that the reduced incidence of atherosclerosis in developing countries is due to the high fibre content of the diet. This evidence was an association, and when it was reported that in experimental animals on high-fibre regimens there was an increased excretion of bile salts, there was a tendency to assume that fibre not only prevents atherosclerosis but does this by increasing the excretion of cholesterol. This assumption may be true, but it is not acceptable on the evidence so far presented, especially as studies in man, unlike those in chicks, rabbits and rats, have as yet failed to find a fall in serum cholesterol concentration on high cereal fibre diets.

It is inherent in any hypothesis that casts its net as wide as does that on fibre, that much of the hypothesis will have to be discarded as new facts are learned. This being so, it is essential that those aspects of the hypothesis which become untenable must be immediately discarded and not perpetuated. Failure to do so could lead to unwarranted therapy, as well as bring into disrepute a hypothesis that contains much that could well be useful.

6 Fibre may help certain conditions but that does not mean it will prevent them

At the moment, it seems that the one clinical condition in which the fibre in the diet is of therapeutic value is diverticulosis. Intraluminal colonic pressure is high in diverticular disease, and gut transit is prolonged, fibre in the form of bran has been shown to reduce both intraluminal pressure and transit time. The patients also have markedly fewer symptoms. In addition, although it is not documented, the softer stools caused by an increased intake of fibre almost certainly ease the discomfort of haemorrhoids and may well contribute to their improvement.

It is not correct, however, to assume that because an agent is therapeutic, the application of that agent, *sine qua non*, prevents the disease arising. It may be that a fibre-rich diet is prophylactic against diverticular disease and haemorrhoids, but to state that because the fibre-rich diet improves these conditions, its deficiency must therefore be a causative agent is not good logic. Aspirin may cure a headache, but a headache is not due to aspirin deficiency.

Another condition where dietary fibre has been shown to be therapeutically useful is in diabetes. Certain types of dietary fibre, by no means the majority, can, when taken with food, reduce the blood glucose and insulin response. It will be noticed that the two clinical situations so far shown to benefit from dietary fibre are in the realm of treatment, not prevention where the main thrust of the health value of fibre lies.

7 Fibre may have harmful side effects

One of the advantages of white flour is that the removal of the husk (bran) means that much of the phytate is removed. It may be that the possible harmful role of phytate in forming an insoluble calcium compound and hence leading to a deficient intake of calcium has been exaggerated, especially in developed countries where calcium tends to be high. However, the recognition that trace amounts of metals such as zinc, chromium, magnesium, and copper are essential in the diet has led to the suggestion that these metals may also form insoluble compounds with phytate. If the intake of these trace elements is low and the small amount consumed is then made unavailable by the phytate in some fibre, a deficiency state may be produced. There is evidence that the presence of fibre in the form of whole wheat has led to iron, calcium and zinc depletion in children in Iran.

Other hazards of dietary fibre that have been suggested are volvulus and intussusception, two abnormal conditions of the small intestine found in the very young, which are fatal without surgical intervention. It is considered that these conditions may be the result of the bulk of its contents, caused by the excessive consumption of vegetable roughage.

These observations obviously need to be substantiated, but they make the point that there are few substances that are consumed that are beneficial under all circumstances to all people, and before recommending an increase in dietary fibre intake, it would be wise to examine its effects carefully and in more depth.

The decrease in transit time (if, indeed this is a property of fibre) leaves less time for the processes of digestion and absorption, and the physicochemical effects of fibre, such as water-binding, may reduce the rate of diffusion of the products of digestion towards the absorption surface. The mechanical erosion of the mucosal surface of the gut could lead to increased losses of endogenous material. Some of these considerations have received support from a study in men and women where it was found that increasing the intake of unavailable carbohydrate (fibre) resulted in a greater fecal loss of energy and in most instances, of nitrogen and fat.

8 The fibre debate – confused definitions and too much speculation

It has been stated earlier that the term dietary fibre means different things to different people, and an attempt has been made to accept a single definition of dietary fibre as 'the remnants of vegetable cell walls that are not hydrolyzed by the alimentary enzymes of man'. Not only must there be international agreement on the definition of fibre, but it must be appreciated that not all dietary fibre has the same composition. Indeed, some dietary fibre, eg wheat-bran, contains, apart from the fibre, several active nutritional ingredients, which themselves can and do influence metabolic activity.

There are statements in the medical literature that the fibre content of the diet has decreased, particularly in Britain since the advent of roller milling in 1880–1890. A more precise assessment of the fibre content of the diet has shown that there has been no such decrease, but that the nature of the fibre has changed. Thus, it is not only important to agree upon a definition of fibre, but it is likely to be clinically more useful if the various components of dietary fibre were studied in isolation. The high speculation-to-fact ratio in the field of dietary fibre could be reduced if careful research with fibre isolates could be carried out, preferably in man.

Many of the preventive health claims made for dietary fibre may be true but it does a discredit to medicine and nutrition should any of these claims subsequently prove to be false.

Notes and References

Carbohydrates in human nutrition, FAO/WHO Report 15, 1980, pp. 55–58.

6 Exploding the Myths About Sugar: The Case of Hypoglycaemia

Vincent Marks

Low blood sugar – the most common misdiagnosed disease (title of book, 1972)
Sugar isn't always sweet (title of book, 1983)
'How sugar starvation became a fashion' (headline of article in *The Times*, 4 November, 1983)

1 More than one sugar

There is no shortage of literature on sugar and its effects upon our health and behaviour. But sugar means different things to different people. To the chemist, sugars are compounds that contain carbon, oxygen and hydrogen (the last two in exactly the same proportions in which they occur in water), hence the alternative name for them of carbohydrates. They range in complexity from small molecules containing only three carbon atoms to giant molecules containing many hundreds. The largest sugars are really a number of smaller sugars joined together in a specific way which determines not only their chemical and physical nature but also their biological importance. Starch and cellulose, for example, are both made up exclusively of glucose units – each containing six carbon atoms – but, as everyone knows, starch is a source of energy when eaten by people, whereas cellulose is not. This is because starch can be broken down by digestive enzymes in the intestines into glucose, which is the only form in which it can be absorbed into the body proper. Cellulose can be broken down but only by certain kinds of bacteria that live in the intestines of animals, such as cows and horses, but not man.

To the medical doctor, speaking in the vernacular, sugar is synonymous with glucose, this being the particular, and only, type of sugar that occurs in the body and which is present in the blood of all of us, as well as in the urine of those who suffer from diabetes. Draft dodgers, who were not aware of this fact, thought they could avoid conscription during the First World War by adding 'sugar', ie sucrose, to their urine when they reported for medical examination. They were however disappointed as the method used to detect glucose in the urine does not detect sucrose which must be broken down in the gut into its constituent parts, namely glucose and another sugar called fructose, before it can be absorbed into the body.

The food industry recognises different grades as well as different types of sugar. These differ both chemically and physically from each other and are often referred to according to their origin, eg milk sugar (lactose), fruit sugar (fructose), corn syrup (a mixture of glucose, maltose and starch hydrolysate). Politicians and farmers distinguish between cane and beet sugar although both are sucrose and chemically identical. To the housewife 'sugar' is synonymous with sucrose and may be 'white' or 'brown', powdered, cubed, granulated or crystallized. Finally to certain self-styled nutritionists – whom I shall more descriptively call food propagandists, since they seem more concerned with publicising themselves than informing the public – sugar is 'natural' or 'added' with the implication, in the context in which these terms are used, that 'natural' is good and 'added' is bad for our health. But chemically 'natural' and 'added' sugars are identical and may be glucose, fructose or, more often, sucrose or a mixture of all three; occasionally sugar may be lactose (milk sugar) which has now become very cheap.

2 Science and nutrition

> 'Carbohydrates, sucrose and human disease', title of article by E.L. Bierman in *American Journal of Clinical Nutrition*, Vol. 3, No. 2, 1979, pp. 2712–2722

The point of this rather long introduction is to emphasise that in order to communicate with each other we must first agree on a common language and understanding of the words used. This can be extremely difficult even for such a comparatively simple subject – chemically speaking – as sugar. How much more difficult then for the whole subject of nutrition; for in the nutrition debate many so-called experts, who have no more authority than that acquired by virtue of the personal life-long usage of food, feel entitled to expound their prejudices as facts. In the communications business (Table 1) – which I have likened to the game of Chinese Whispers – such individuals have the edge over scientists insofar as they do not have to waste their time doing experiments and making observations which can be validated (but which are the true basis of all our knowledge). They can instead rely upon selected anecdotes to convey their message or just use their imagination. Skilfully presented anecdotes are more intelligible to the public than the rather dull reports used by scientists to communicate with one another. In such reports scientists carefully distinguish between their observations and results, and their interpretations of them. Others may interpret the same facts – providing they are established as facts – differently from the original authors; sometimes more correctly because of the additional information they possess.

Table 1: Sources of Information on Nutrition

Sources	*Type of author*	*Type of publication*	
Primary	Scientists and epidemiologists	Original research papers in "peer reviewed" journals	
Secondary	Scientists	Reviews and monographs	
Tertiary	Academic authors and expert panels	Text-books and "consensus" reports	
Quaternary	Popularists	"Popular" books	
Quinternary	Journalists	Popular Magazines, newspaper articles, television and radio presentations.	
Sexternary	Copy-writers	Advertisements and PR handouts	FOLKLORE
Septernary	Food-propagandists	Statements and press interviews	CUSTOMS

My own involvement with nutrition in general, and with the nutritional aspects of sugar in particular, has been as a clinical scientist who, because his observations and research brought him into conflict with the unsubstantiated opinions of the food propagandists, found himself embroiled in what he takes to be a complex politico-economic debate which has very little to do with clinical or medical science on the one hand, or the public good on the other. Mud-slinging or the impugning of motives of persons with differing views is all grist to the mill. For a taste of the debate, consider the following passage which appeared in an article by Annabel Ferriman, headed 'New Food Labels Anger Doctors', (*The Observer*, 26th May 1985):

> Four influential health and consumer groups insist however that the carbohydrate content should not appear without the sugar content. The

Health Education Council, the Coronary Prevention Group, the Consumers Association and the British Dietetic Association are all expected to demand such a change. It is uncertain whether their combined power can combat the influence of the sugar industry with its Westminster Lobbyists. The director of the Sugar Bureau is Michael Shersby, Conservative MP for Uxbridge, while Mr. Colin Moynihan, Parliamentary Private Secretary to Health Minister Kenneth Clarke is Chief Executive of Ridgeways Tea, a wholly-owned subsidiary of Tate and Lyle.

3 Sugar – 'toxicologically safe and nutritionally acceptable'

Sucrose, commonly known as table sugar, cane sugar, or beet sugar is one of few organic compounds which play an important role in human nutrition, available in large quantities of high purity at a relatively low cost; it is the standard of naturally occurring sweetness, joining other nutrients usually carbohydrate in nature that comprise a group of palatable foodstuffs known to be relatively efficient sources of energy, simple in composition and rapidly metabolisable for utilisation and storage in the body. It is a compound toxicologically safe and nutritionally acceptable. Its direct intake in normal amounts should be recommendable to all healthy populations; its use in processed foods should be controlled to ensure that adverse effects would not occur from deficiencies as well as from excesses in nutrient intake. Its use should be balanced with other carbohydrate constituents. (From a paper on 'The Development of Sugar Substitutes; a comparative toxicological and nutritional overview, by G. Vettorazzi, Toxicologist at the World Health Organisation, Geneva).

I recently came across the notes I made for a talk on the nutritional aspects of sugar given at a public meeting some 11 years ago. I concluded then, as now, that 'there is very little convincing evidence that increased consumption of sugar (sucrose) is really responsible, in the population as a whole, for producing any disease apart from caries of the teeth...' I was reported, however, as saying that sugar in the diet causes disease.

Once it ceased being a luxury because of its high cost, sugar enjoyed a well-deserved reputation among the general public as one of the good things of life. It not only made many otherwise unpleasant foods palatable, but provided a ready and cheap source of energy, especially for those engaged in heavy manual work and active children with naturally high metabolic rates. It also served as the basis of dietary delicacies we refer to collectively as confectionery. How then has it now come about that sugar, at best, is thought of as 'naughty but nice' or, as it was recently described by a professor of dentistry in a television programme on food, as a 'toxin'. This must surely be a gross misuse of the English language and I cannot but think the speaker deliberately meant to mislead his audience. But it shows how enthusiasm can cause even the knowledgeable to present their opinions as facts.

There has always been a core of detractors who have objected to the use of sugar. Their grounds were mainly socio-economic or puritanical, eg anti-slave traders or anti-colonialists, but some believed it was unhealthy. This is the tack now adopted by the detractors who claim to speak as 'nutritionists' and make it necessary to re-examine the validity of their arguments and, if found wanting, expose them as fraudulent.

4 The questionable basis of the arguments against sugar

> *The Saccharine Disease; conditions caused by the taking of refined carbohydrates, such as Sugar and White Flour,* title of book by T. L. Cleave

The argument that sugar in the diet is a major factor in the causation of a number of what are often emotively, but meaninglessly, referred to as diseases of affluence stems largely from the publication by Cleave. He considered a number of well-known conditions amongst which he included obesity, diabetes, diverticular disease of the colon, varicose veins, gall bladder disease, coronary heart disease and dental caries, to be but various manifestations of the dietary consequences of eating not only sugar but also refined white flour. He did not consider sugar (sucrose) any more harmful than white flour. The emphasis upon sugar as the culprit – if indeed there is a culprit at all – must therefore be placed at the feet of others of less perception than Cleave, who was amongst the first in modern times to appreciate the true importance of dietary fibre.

Many of the diseases, eg, dental caries and obesity, said to be caused by sugar in the diet are dealt with elsewhere in this volume. I will not discuss them further except to reiterate the views expressed earlier that, with the exception of dental caries, the evidence implicating sugar (sucrose) in their causation is flimsy, to say the least, and on a par with that implied by the question 'When did you stop beating your wife?' In other words, those such as myself who believe that,used in moderation, sugar has a useful role to play in modern nutrition, are expected to prove that it (sucrose) is not the cause of obesity, coronary heart disease or what you will, whilst the detractors just allege that it is.

5 Does sugar cause hyperactivity and crime?

> The root of crime can lie in childhood hyperactivity. New research shows that hyperactivity, delinquency and criminal behaviour can be caused by processed, junk food, heavy in fat, salt and – especially – sugar. (Part of preamble to an article by Barbara Rigg, *New Health*, December 1983)

Recently sugar has been designated by the food propagandists as a major causative factor in behavioural problems in adults and children, ranging in severity from mild and only minimally inconvenient to habitual delinquency and recidivism. This suggestion, like others linking sugar usage with various diseases, is based on unjustified extrapolation from epidemiological and experimental data, if on anything at all, and is totally at variance with the facts as determined by proper controlled clinical trials and observations. The idea that sugar (sucrose) might cause delinquency and other types of abnormal behaviour would gain credibility, despite the large body of negative evidence against it, if a realistic causative mechanism could be postulated and critically examined.

6 Hypoglycaemia (low blood sugar)

> 'Diet away your stress, tension and anxiety; a new commonsense plan for the control of low blood sugar related disorders, including overeating and obesity, migraine headaches, alcoholism, mental disturbances, hypoglycaemia and hyperactivity'. (Extract from dust cover of a book by J. Daniel Palm, 1976)

Virtually the only mechanism proposed to explain the postulated link between sugar (sucrose) ingestion and behavioural disorders is the belief that sugar in the diet predisposes to the development of a condition known as hypoglycaemia – which literally means low blood sugar (ie, glucose). Hypoglycaemia is universally accepted by medical practitioners as being capable, when it occurs, of causing aberrant behaviour even in the most staid and law-abiding citizen. It is, however, extremely rare, except in patients overtreated with insulin. In order to explain how hypoglycaemia is caused and how it affects behaviour, it is necessary to become somewhat technical.

As mentioned at the beginning of this chapter, glucose is the only type of sugar that occurs in the body, no matter in what form sugar (including starch) is eaten in the food. In other words, the body itself – mainly the intestines and liver – converts all sugars in the diet into glucose before it allows them to enter the bloodstream. Glucose cannot be stored in the body as such, but must be turned into animal starch or glycogen which can be deposited in the liver for use when energy requirements are not being met by the absorption of glucose from the intestine. Normally the body controls the amount of sugar (glucose) in the blood within very narrow limits by independently adjusting the rates at which glucose is put into or removed from deposit – just like a well-run current account at the bank. If for any reasons these rates get out of step, the blood glucose may rise too high – producing a condition we recognise as diabetes or hyperglycaemia – or too low – giving rise to hypoglycaemia. Hypoglycaemia, unlike diabetes, cannot be tolerated for more than very short periods and manifests itself by malfunction of the brain.

The brain, unlike virtually all of the other organs of the body, depends exclusively upon glucose brought to it in the bloodstream for its energy needs and to enable it to work properly. So important is it for the economy of the body to maintain blood sugar (glucose) levels above the minimum necessary to keep the brain working properly that there are many reserve mechanisms that can be brought into play whenever the supply of sugar (glucose) to the brain is threatened. These mechanisms cut down the expenditure or usage of sugar (glucose) by other tissues, by encouraging them to burn fat instead, and also mobilise the reserve stores of sugar (glycogen) in the liver. This defence mechanism can be impaired when insulin, the hormone used to treat diabetes, ie high blood sugar (glucose), is inadvertently given in too high a dose. Insulin works both by increasing utilisation (expenditure) of glucose in the tissues, and by reducing its withdrawal from liver stores. Hypoglycaemia can also occur as an unwelcome complication in a number of extremely rare diseases in which case it is usually referred to as 'spontaneous hypoglycaemia' to distinguish it from iatrogenic, ie, doctor-induced, hypoglycaemia.

Proper use of insulin in patients with diabetes ensures that the blood sugar (glucose) falls from abnormally high to normal levels. However, if too much insulin is used, the mechanism that normally protects the body against the development of a low blood sugar level may be overwhelmed and the brain is temporarily deprived of its energy supply and consequently malfunctions. Amongst the manifestations of this type of brain malfunction are the appearance of various unpleasant symptoms and, in a tiny proportion of cases, aberrant behaviour including a tendency to become obstreperous or even violent. These symptoms and behaviour patterns are, however, common in the general population and are by no means specific to hypoglycaemia. This cause should only be considered, therefore, when the blood glucose concentration is *measurably* low and the symptoms and behavioural abnormalities are completely and specifically reversed by sugar (starch, sucrose or glucose) given by mouth or glucose given by intravenous injection, and by nothing else.

7 Misdiagnoses of hypoglycaemia

> 'Non-hypoglycemia is an epidemic condition' (title of article by J. Yager and R.T. Young in *The New England Journal of Medicine*, October 1974, p.907)

There are a large number of practitioners, mostly of alternative or fringe medicine, who diagnose hypoglycaemia on the flimsiest of evidence which seldom includes a measurement of the blood glucose concentration at the relevant time. If they do bother to measure the blood glucose concentration at all, they do so only during the course of a so-called prolonged glucose tolerance test, the use of which in the diagnosis of 'spontaneous hypoglycaemia' has long been discredited. A diagnosis of 'hypoglycaemia' made under these circumstances is usually incorrect but is socially acceptable, whereas alternative and, in many cases more truthful, diagnoses such as inadequate personality, neurosis, psychopathy or even chronic alcohol abuse, are not. The favoured treatment for this spurious condition is to 'correct' the purported dietary abnormalities that cause it. Chief amongst these is said to be the presence of 'added' or 'hidden' sugar (sucrose) in the diet. This has therefore to be rigorously excluded. Additional treatments include vitamins – usually in large doses – sold at inflated prices by the very people who have prescribed them – and, until recently, a worthless nostrum called adrenocortical extract (ACE). This extract was claimed to be necessary to correct a postulated deficient action of the patients' own adrenal glands.

Concern over extensive misdiagnosis prompted the following warning in the United States:

> Recent publicity in the popular press has led the public to believe that there is a widespread and unrecognised occurrence of hypoglycemia in this country. Furthermore it has been suggested repeatedly that the condition is causing many of the symptoms that affect the American population. These claims are not supported by medical evidence. Because of the possible widespread misunderstanding about the matter, three organisations of physicians and scientists (The American Diabetes Association, The Endocrine Society, and the American

> Medical Association) have issued this statement concerning diagnosis and treatment of hypoglycemia. (Introductory remarks to a Statement on Hypoglycemia, *Diabetes*, No.22, 1973, p.137)

8 Hypoglycaemia and criminality

> In 1977, a US Senate Select Committee on Nutrition and Human Needs, heard an Ohio probation officer, Mrs. Barbara Reed, testify to her success in treating offenders by diet. The offenders were tested for hypoglyacemia with a written questionnaire. She found a high proportion of the people she questioned appeared to be hypoglycaemic but responded remarkably well to being placed on a diet to correct the condition: no sugar, coffee, alcohol, sweets, or processed food containing additives. (Extract from article entitled 'Sugar's Bitter Harvest', *The Times*, 1st August, 1983.)

Whatever effects the warning by the tripartite bodies may or may not have had upon the American sick, it did not prevent the exploitation of 'hypoglycaemia' by social workers and criminologists. They promoted it as a cause – indeed the most important cause in some people's eyes – of delinquency and criminal behaviour amongst young people. So persuasive were some of these individuals that, despite the complete absence of scientifically acceptable evidence as to the correctness of their views, the judiciaries in some communities imposed penalties upon juvenile offenders which included compulsory participation in certain dietary regimes.

> By 1975 one of the judges was already instructing defendants – "Mrs. Reed is going to put you on a diet and you will stay on it or you will go to jail because you will be back in trouble if you go off it..." (Extract from 'Sugar's Bitter Harvest', *The Times*, 1st August, 1983)

I have a copy of *Back to Basics*, a booklet written by Mrs. Reed and two judges, which is subtitled 'How one probation officer uses nutrition to improve health and maintain the attention of clients referred by the court'. It accepts as fact the very material that the tripartite bodies warned against as quackery only a few years earlier.

Some penal institutions in the USA have gone so far as to make adjustments to the composition of the food they provide for their inmates or permit them to eat. These adjustments are made on the basis of advice given to them by self-appointed nutritionists whose authority does not derive from any fundamental research in nutrition but comes instead from experiments which are flawed in design and over-interpreted. The studies best known in this country are those of S.J. Schoenthaler, a criminologist from California who described them in a little-known publication *The International Journal of Biosocial Research*. This journal, which is subscribed to by none of the major British libraries, does exist and I personally have a copy obtained on a visit to the USA. This has enabled me to evaluate Schoenthaler's work with the same thoroughness I would apply to any other investigator but it does not explain how the many journalists and other nutrition propagandists who have written so enthusiastically about it in this country obtained their information.

The popularists have, almost without exception, failed to mention – far less draw attention to the fact – that of the five studies carried out by Schoenthaler, the first four purported to show a reduction of violent behaviour in young male inmates of penal institutions when they were fed a low sugar (sucrose) diet. The fifth study showed exactly the opposite, namely a reduction in violent behaviour in the inmates whose diet contained more sugar (sucrose, fructose, glucose) than the control group, achieved by adding 'orange juice with no additives nor added sugar' to their ordinary diet. I wonder if this is because the apologists have never read the original publications or because they failed to appreciate that orange juice contains the same sugar, ie sucrose, as comes out of a packet, in addition to glucose and fructose. Whatever the reason, I suspect that unwelcome facts would not be allowed to interfere with a good story, namely that sugar makes delinquents out of decent, well-brought-up children and thugs out of their older brothers and sisters.

The diet theory of malevolence which exonerates both the parents and those responsible for the administration of the social environment in which the delinquents have grown up, is eminently press-worthy. It has a superficial resemblance to the theory that considers alcoholism to be a disease. Unlike the latter theory, however, it has absolutely no foundation in fact, at least in its present form which has all the features of searching for and finding a scapegoat in the shape of sugar (sucrose).

> Cola contains seven spoonfuls of sugar per glass and it is more than likely that it is this which caused the riots in Brixton and the North when the very hot weather would have sent the consumption of cola right up and with it overdosing of the blood sugar, hence creating hypoglycaemia which creates a violent nature. (Extract from a letter to *The Surrey Advertiser*, April 1984)

9 Hyperactivity in children not caused by sugar

> Therefore the panel concluded that at the present time there is no acceptable evidence to support a causal relationship between sugar intake and behavioural disturbances or to justify changes in public policy (eg alterations of diet plans in schools, correction facilities or other institutions) based on this claim. (Extract from 'Statement of the Resource Conference on Diet and Behaviour', *Nutrition Reviews*, No.42, 1984, p.200)

Whilst hyperactivity in children does exist as a clinical entity it is undoubtedly rare, if strict diagnostic criteria are adhered to – which, unfortunately, is seldom the case. The idea, strongly promoted in the USA, especially California, the eastern seaboard of Australia and, increasingly, in Britain, that 'hyperactivity' in children is common and due to sugar in the diet, allergy to food additives, and/or a combination of the two, has no scientific support and is contrary to the experimental evidence. In a tiny percentage of cases hyperactivity may be associated with genuine, specific and confirmable allergy to one or more food constituents (not including sucrose). These are just as likely to be normal ingredients of the diet, such as cows' milk, as chemically defined additives. Most children to whom the diagnosis of 'hyperactivity' is attached are, however, neither suffering from hyperactivity nor food allergies but from parents or teachers who are unable to cope with them. Hyperactivity, like hypoglycaemia and, unlike alternative explanations, is a socially acceptable condition.

10 Many of the new dietary authoritarians not experts

The authoritarianism we have witnessed in regard to what is or is not a suitable diet for behaviour control is spreading into other areas. There are already those who, on just as flimsy evidence as exists in relation to sugar and disease, are ready, whenever the opportunity arises, to impose their views on what constitutes a healthy diet upon others – by legislation if necessary. They have fervour instead of knowledge and suffer the malady of the ignorant which is to be ignorant of their own ignorance. To extrapolate from epidemiological data – as many of those who bother about data at all often do – to forecast the likely outcome of an enforced food policy is unscientific and potentially dangerous both socially and medically.

How can we distinguish genuine nutritionists – of whom there undoubtedly are some – from the self-appointed nutritionists or 'pseuds'? One of the simplest ways is to examine their language. Pseuds refer to 'junk food' without defining what it is or why it is junk; they talk of 'added' or 'hidden' sugar, of 'healthy foods', *brown* sugar, *white* sugar and *raw* sugar instead of just sugar. They speak of 'hypoglycaemia' as though it was a disease in its own right instead of being a complication of one. They advocate analysis of hair for trace elements, and vitamin and trace element supplements even when there is no evidence that they are required. Pseuds are unaware of the ill effects of excessive vitamin and mineral intake; above all, they have no research publications describing their own original observations, or experiments in the reputable international, refereed scientific literature. They do however have the ear of the sensationalist media, especially that which subscribes to the anti-scientific approach exemplified by the statement:

> 'Scientists are the last people to understand anything, they have as much chance of finding truth in a test tube as in a crystal ball...' (taken from a statement by Teddy Goldsmith in *The Sunday Times* Colour Supplement, 1985)

If the purpose and nature of science is so poorly understood by opinion-formers such as Teddy Goldsmith, perhaps the time has come for them to emerge from their laboratories and speak to the public directly instead of through impressionable popularists who seemingly cannot distinguish good from bad evidence.

7 Dental Caries and the Conscientious Consumer

Marshall Midda

1 Conventional dental health rules about sugar and frequent visits to the dentist

Dental decay is an ancient disease affecting man long before there were any processed foods containing refined carbohydrates such as sucrose. During the last decade, over 200 million pounds has been spent on world caries research. The end result has been a sharp decrease in the incidence of dental decay and in the United Kingdom, studies have shown not only reduced caries prevalence but in addition they have demonstrated an increase in the number of decay-free individuals. There has been an improvement in oral health at a time when there has been no major change, or, if anything, an increase in the use of sugar or other carbohydrates. This vast amount of research has also demonstrated that the caries process is not yet completely understood.

There is also mounting world evidence that conventional repair visits to the dentist are no guarantee that teeth can be kept for life. The old rules for dental health namely, brush after every meal, don't eat sweets and visit the dentist every six months, are now shown to be scientifically incorrect. These traditional patterns of repair and prevention would now seem to fail patients. Perpetuation of antiquated dental myths is counter-productive to the health interests of the British public. It would be a pity if reliance upon traditional dental science continues to endorse beliefs and practices which could well have a negative dental health impact upon people. Consumers have a right to a more sophisticated knowledge on the whole subject and especially the relationship between caries and nutrition.

2 Changing theories in caries formation

In order for the carious process to occur there must be several factors present. Obviously there must be a tooth, but it must be one that is susceptible to decay and that depends on features such as heredity, social and racial background, nutrition of the tooth before, during and after eruption and the level of fluoride incorporated within the enamel as well as at the surface of the tooth.

Contrary to popular belief, decay is not primarily a dietary disease, but one of microbial origin. There must be bacteria in the form of mature dental plaque, which can be defined as a soft, bacterial deposit which forms on teeth not adequately cleaned. The older and thicker the plaque film, the greater the levels of acid that can be produced.

Dietary elements do have an important role in that the bacteria need food and take their metabolic needs from a vast range of foodstuffs, not just sucrose. The micro-organisms which are firmly adherent to the tooth, absorb and breakdown carbohydrates, releasing organic acids and other noxious waste products onto the tooth and its supporting structures causing decay and gum disease.

Caries is not instantaneous, it needs considerable time. A tooth in someone susceptible to decay which was not cleaned or cared for in any way, would take many months before it showed any signs of caries. Time is dependant upon the retention of the food on the teeth as well as the frequency with which it is taken. In addition saliva modifies all of the previous factors and has the ability with fluoride to help repair the damaged enamel.

3 The features of fluoride

Dental decay is not a simple dissolution of the tooth surface by bacterial acid, as formerly thought. Many researchers now feel that the formation of a carious lesion is the result of a dynamic series of events rather than continuing acid attack. The initial lesion appears as a demineralisation beneath the tooth surface. The means of entry of the hydrogen ions (acid) into the sub-surface zone and means of exit of the products of demineralisation are not fully understood. In addition to demineralisation, periods of remineralisation occur in which mineral ions are deposited from saliva into the affected areas. Dental caries begins when the duration and intensity of the demineralisation exceeds that of the remineralisation phase. Epidemiological studies have demonstrated the disappearance, or clinical 'healing' of carious lesions as long as they are only within the enamel. When fluoride is present at the tooth surface, it favours remineralisation. This dynamic process is affected by a variety of factors, including proteins, organic acids and amino acids present in plaque fluid. It has also been demonstrated that it is the complex salivary proteins which favour and control the demineralisation phase, and fluoride favours the remineralisation phase. Fluoride interferes with the metabolic enzymatic pathways of the bacteria and during demineralisation the released fluoride ions help form insoluble calcium fluoride and thus prevent further mineral loss. Caries can thus be referred to as a *fluoride-deficiency disease*. Caries is multifactorial. All the aetiological agents have to be present and the removal of any one of these factors would result in the absence of decay.

4 Diet and decay

Diet influences caries in two ways, either by inhibiting or promoting the disease. Far more attention has been paid to the latter rather than the former influence. In recent years the area of greatest controversy has been that of the role of sugar in the caries process and an attempt to control caries by recommending abstention.

The principal dietary causative factor in caries formation is the consumption of *any* and *all* fermentable carbohydrates, which include milk, fruits and honey. Whatever and whenever people eat, they are likely to consume some fermentable carbohydrate, thus exposing their teeth to a cariogenic challenge. Research has been performed on the mechanics of caries formation, on efforts to determine the potential cariogenicity of natural and processed foodstuffs and on epidemiological efforts to correlate dietary patterns with caries incidence. The results of these investigations have indicated that continued usage of the simplistic traditional advice, the only apparent goal of which was to limit sugar consumption, as a basis for public policy recommendations may be considered as endorsing outdated and misleading interpretations of the relationship between carbohydrate consumption and caries formation.

5 Blaming sugar in processed foods as the most cariogenic substance is specious

There is a popular belief that a decrease in consumption of certain processed food products containing sugars will reduce or eliminate tooth decay. Breakfast cereals, confectionery and soft drinks are the usual targets of such thinking.

Current research findings employing animal, human and in vitro testing methods all attempted to assess the relative cariogenicity of the same test foods and confectionery products. In all three participating laboratories and in all three test methods used, the findings indicated that unsweetened wheat flakes and biscuits were more cariogenic than pure sucrose.

In seeking to establish (in both animals and humans) the relative cariogenicity of various foods compared to sucrose it was found in recent research funded by the National Institute for Dental Research and the Food and Drug Administration that when starches are combined with sucrose, the resulting combinations of food are often as much as twice as potentially cariogenic as when sucrose is used alone. Conversely, many individual foods and combinations of foods have been shown to affect the cariogenic potential of the diet. For example, the combination of sucrose with such foods as peanuts or cheese emerges as potentially less cariogenic than sucrose alone. Research conducted by the Forsyth Institute indicated that chocolate exhibits properties that offset the cariogenicity of sucrose. It also remarked that in its cariogenicity experiments 'a few snacks with high sugar content exhibited only moderate cariogenic potential'.

It must be remembered that there are no animal or human tests, singly or in combination, in vivo or in vitro, which have been recognised as scientifically probative of the relative cariogenicity of foodstuffs. Thus there is no current scientific basis for categorical statements concerning the potential relative cariogenicity in humans of sugars or foods containing fermentable carbohydrates. It is frequency of carbohydrate consumption, rather than the amount of sugar consumed, which is the major dietary determinant of caries causation.

6 All fermentable carbohydrates are potentially cariogenic

An example of misinformation was the 1980 dietary guideline published by the US Department of Agriculture which advised consumers that 'jams, jellies, candies, cookies, soft drinks, cakes, pies, breakfast cereals, catsup, flavoured milks and ice cream' were the villains in dental decay and urged consumers to 'select fresh fruits' instead.

This was confusing and misleading since within the broad spectrum of unprocessed 'natural' foods there exists a substantial sugar content every bit as potentially cariogenic as processed foodstuffs containing added sugars. Dr. Sanford Miller, director of the FDA's Centre for Food Safety and Applied Nutrition stated

> Most consumers believe that it is added sugar that is cariogenic and should be controlled rather than accepting the fact that, to the oral flora, all simple sugars, are fuel for the mill. Thus, dates, figs and honey are equally if not more cariogenic than sugar-coated cereals. To the public, however, if the good Lord put it there it must be alright.

Responding to an inquiry from the US senate, the NIDR stated in 1983 that:

> Naturally sweet foods such as raisins, figs and apples have high sugar content and are presumably cariogenic if frequently eaten...We strongly advise the public to avoid frequent ingestion of unprocessed foods – raisins for example – that have a high sugar content.

In 1983, Bibby exposed the potential damage from the sugars and natural acids found in unprocessed fruits and vegetables, and in addition demonstrated the cariogenic potential of bread. From this and other work it can now be shown that dentally the most dangerous foods may be those which contain combinations of cooked starches and sugars (for example, cakes, pies and bread) rather than merely sugars themselves.

After careful deliberation and reconsideration, in the spring of 1985 the US Department of Agriculture revised its guidelines to inform consumers that starches as well as sugars are potentially cariogenic.

In addition, three of the American Dental Association's Councils (the Councils on Dental Health and Health Planning, Dental Research and Dental Therapeutics) issued a joint Statement on Diet and Caries. It declared:

> Sucrose has traditionally been regarded as the carbohydrate most detrimental to teeth. Evidence indicates, however, that cariogenic bacteria can use other simple carbohydrates to produce acid in the mouth. These include corn sweeteners and some other sweeteners that may be added to processed foods, as well as fructose and glucose, which occur naturally in honey, fruits and some vegetables. Some research suggests that even foods that contain more complex carbohydrates (starches) may have the potential to promote caries...
>
> The Association recognises that the single action of decreasing total sucrose intake may be incomplete as a caries preventive measure. Many foods that contain little or no sucrose, but that do contain other fermentable carbohydrates are capable of promoting decay.

Thus any proposed British legislation on nutritional labelling which attempted to show the sugar content separately from the total carbohydrates present would not only be misleading but also incorrect in terms of dental health, since the other carbohydrates present are equally if not more involved in the caries process.

7 The amount of sugar does not determine relative cariogenicity
Findings indicate that the amount of sucrose in a foodstuff does not determine its potential cariogenicity. There is no evidence today to support the contention that the cariogenic potential of a foodstuff is a function of its sucrose content. Imfeld et al. demonstrated that a one per cent sucrose solution changes the acid in human plaque to the same degree as do five and ten per cent sucrose solutions. Other workers have shown that cultures of cariogenic organisms can thrive at sucrose content percentage levels as low as 0.5 per cent.

In animal experimentation, researchers have attempted to determine the relationship of the amount of dietary sucrose to caries formation. It has been shown that increasing the sucrose content in a rat's diet from five per cent to 15 per cent does not increase the caries experience. Other tests found it necessary to reduce the percentage of dietary sucrose from 67 per cent down to between four per cent and eight per cent before any caries reduction could be observed, and the maximum caries challenge in rats was obtained at sucrose levels as low as three per cent.

The important subject of the relationship between amount of sucrose intake and caries incidence was discussed at the Food, Nutrition and Dental Health Conference sponsored by the American Dental Association in 1978. It was reported that a reduction of as much as 25 per cent of the sucrose content in foods such as cakes, confectionery, jelly and pies produced no measurable caries reduction.

8 Carbohydrates and energy
Any discussion of diet and dental caries must proceed with the awareness that everyone needs a certain carbohydrate intake in order to sustain life, and that all carbohydrates can cause dental caries. There is a marked 'Alice in Wonderland' attitude in urging people to 'use less sugar' and to 'eat less of foods containing sugar', since this implies that (a) people can live without sugars, (b) products containing sugars are nutritionally undesirable and (c) there exists a realistic and safe spectrum of alternatives to such sugar-containing foods.

Carbohydrates are commonly divided into two sub-groups, sugars and starches, the distinction is simply one of form. The sugars are composed of mono- or di-saccharides which are substances composed of one or two molecule sugar units. The starches can be considered as complex sugars since they consist of multi-molecule glucose sugar units, and are described as polysaccharides.

Fermentable carbohydrates are ubiquitous in common processed and 'natural' foods for a good biological reason – each living cell requires energy simply to maintain its basic internal life processes and carbohydrates are a vital source of that energy. The body's primary fuel during activity is glucose which is the basic nutrient end product derived from the digestion and absorption of all carbohydrate foods, whether starches or sugars, processed or 'natural'.

In 1977 the Council for Agricultural Science and Technology recommended in its Dietary Goals for the United States that carbohydrate consumption be increased to represent 55 to 60 per cent of total energy intake. If dentists urge reductions in sugar consumption, what are the alternative noncariogenic energy-providing foodstuffs? Presumably, no one would urge increasing fat consumption. Apart from the issue of low energy content, there are few low cost, high protein and low fat foodstuffs which have a wider consumer appeal. There is an understandable limit to the amount of cottage cheese which an individual is willing to eat.

In its 1983 publication *Diet and Dental Health*, the American Dental Association stated:

> You may be wondering if you should simply eliminate all foods that contain sugars from your diet. That wouldn't be a good idea. Your body needs the nutrients found in milk, fruit, vegetables and other foods as well as the calories many of these foods provide. For good dental health, you should learn to use foods that contain sugars wisely, not cut them out of your diet altogether.

9 Dental decay: disease in decline

Epidemiological studies demonstrate that the prevalence of caries in children living in most of the Western civilisations has dramatically decreased during the past 12 years and is continuing to do so. During this time, the per capita consumption of sugar and other carbohydrates has remained fairly constant, any move tending towards an increase.

In 1983 the Robert Wood Johnson Foundation published the results of a five year, $10 million study which indicated that 'a substantial proportion of children had no caries at all' and that 'some 20 per cent of the children accounted for nearly 60 per cent of all decay found'. Dr. Harald Loe, Director of the National Institute of Dental Research, stated in 1983 to the U.S. Senate:

> After centuries of steady increases, tooth decay is now showing a drastic decline. More children are caries free.... It has been estimated that the reduction in caries alone has reduced the Nation's total dental care

> bill for 1981 by two billion dollars.... This reduction in caries prevalence, we believe, is primarily the result of the last two decades of research on caries prevention in general and the effect of fluorides in particular.

In response to questions as to whether it was a reduction in sugar consumption which had led to the demonstrated drop in the incidence of dental caries in the US, the NIDR, unequivocally stated to the Senate that:

> The effect of [substitute sweeteners] on caries prevalence would not have been reflected in recent epidemiological surveys... we do not attribute changes seen thus far to be the result of research on the modification of causative factors in the diet.

The NIDR now indicates that it no longer considers efforts to change eating habits as an effective method of combatting dental decay and does not support programmes which attempt to modify dietary content or behaviour. The results of the National Preventive Dentistry Demonstration Programme sponsored by the Robert Wood Johnson Foundation confirm that educational efforts to alter the diet were the least effective means of reducing tooth decay.

10 Changing the Susceptibility of the Tooth

Of all the factors that can affect the susceptibility of the tooth, the most effective preventive agent is fluoride and it is the acceptance of fluoridated toothpastes by the public that accounts for the recent decline in caries. However, it is well known that systemic and topical fluorides and dietary modifications have a less profound caries preventive effect on the pit and fissure tooth surfaces than on smooth surfaces. These pits and fissures are found primarily on the occlusal or chewing surfaces of molars and premolars. Surveys show that as much as 84 per cent of the dental caries seen in children that do have decay is in these sites. The World Health Organisation's goal for dental health by the Year 2000 is to have less than three decayed, missing or filled teeth. Today, the major remaining need in the youth population is to reduce or eliminate the carious process in pits and fissures. This can be achieved by placing a plastic coating called a fissure sealant onto the vulnerable surfaces of newly erupted teeth. At present this preventive procedure is not allowed under the regulations of the General Dental Services of the National Health Service.

To fail to recommend to the public that they use a combination of fluoride and sealants or to misdirect their attention toward ineffective, incomplete or incorrect dietary suggestions would have the effect of moving dental science decades backwards.

For those individuals who are most susceptible to dental decay, frequency of eating is the main factor. Fermentable carbohydrates may be eaten by the vast majority of the population, who have little or no decay, with little risk. However, those who do easily develop cavities should confine eating to meal times.

11 New guidelines for dental health

From a review of all the current data on the aetiology, prevention and treatment of dental caries, the time is ripe to offer new advice on dental care based upon modern evidence. The suggested guidelines are:

Remove plaque from each surface of each tooth at least once a day. This is different from brushing your teeth; this is cleaning your teeth and gums. Using the right type of toothbrush in the right sort of way, dental floss to clean between the teeth and the occasional use of a disclosing tablet to indicate any plaque left behind will prevent gum disease and help reduce decay.

Fortify with Fluoride. Every day and at every age a fluoride supplement should be used to prevent and heal carious lesions. This may be obtained from many sources including the use of dentrifices, mouth rinses and tablets. To reach those people who are unable to purchase oral hygiene aids, the most cost effective method is by the public water supply. In addition the use of fissure sealants is recommended to protect susceptible surfaces unaffected by fluoride.

Avoid frequent snacking. Good nutritional health is compatible with dental health. The various forms of fermentable carbohydrates can be used as long as there is a clean tooth with a lowered susceptibility. It is better to have larger meals including sugars rather than constant snacking.

Visit the Dentist for a Health Check. There is no magic in the six month recall. Admittedly it is a convenient interval but there are many patients who only need to be seen every two years whilst others may have to be seen at shorter intervals. The role of the patient is altering and instead of being the passive object in the dental chair, it is now the responsibility of the consumers to look after their own mouths and have lower treatment costs. Thus a visit to the dentist is to check that the patient is maintaining his or her own dental health, rather than a crisis or unnecessary situation.

Although it would appear that these new guidelines are more or less the same as the old rules, they are placed in a different and deliberate order, because they relate to what people are most likely to do in a practical world. With the correct use of the information now available to us it can be possible for people to keep their teeth for life.

Notes and References

American Dental Association Statement on diet and caries, *Journal of the American Dental Association*, No. 107, 1983, p.78.

B.G. Bibby, 'Fruits and Vegetables and Dental Caries', *Clinical Preventive Dentistry*, No. 6, 1983, pp.3–11.

T. Imfeld, R. Hirsch, H.R. Muehlmann, 'Telemetric Recordings of Interdental Plaque pH During Different Meal Patterns', *British Dental Journal*, No. 144, 1978, pp.40–43.

M. Midda, 'Clinical Prevention of Dental Caries: The Scientific Basis for Adults', *Journal of the Irish Dental Association*, No. 26, 1980, pp.59–61.

S. Miller, 'Sugar, Oral Health and Regulation' in *Foods, Nutrition and Dental Health*, American Dental Association Health Foundation, 1978, pp.389–391.

National Institute of Dental Health, Budget Request, Testimony before the Senate Committee on Appropriations, 11th April, 1983, pp.645–669.

8 Obesity and the Plumpness Which Needs No Diet

Reg Passmore

1 Obesity a 'serious problem'

Orthodox teaching as set out in medical textbooks is that obesity is a condition that predisposes to many disorders. Of these the most important are high blood pressure (hypertension) and diabetes; both of these are very prevalent in the United Kingdom and other countries with an ample food supply and each is responsible for much chronic ill health and many premature deaths. Treatment of obesity depends upon dietary changes which reduce the energy intake and in most patients an increase in physical activity is both desirable and possible. Many patients find it difficult to break long-established habits and to make the necessary changes in their life-style. Obesity is thus a serious disorder and the best account of it is a book written by Dr. J.S. Garrow, Head of the Nutrition Research Group, Northwick Park Hospital, Harrow, with the title *Treat Obesity Seriously*. I have only one major point of dissent from the views expressed in this excellent book and this is on the criteria used to define and grade obesity.

2 But how fat is obese?

Body weight by itself is not a reliable means of telling whether an individual is or is not obese, nor does it provide a reliable method of grading the extent of obesity. Many different standards which take into account weight, height, body build and estimates of total body fat have been used. There is now a consensus, with which I agree, that the most practical standard is the ratio of weight to the square of height, W/H^2. This is often referred to as the body mass index, not a meaningful scientific term, and it is better to call the ratio Quetelet's Index after the Belgian sociologist who first used it in 1869.

Garrow defines three grades of obesity based on Quetelet's Index, with weight (W) in kilogrammes and height (H) in metres.

Grade III W/H^2 >40
Grade II W/H^2 30–40
Grade I W/H^2 25–29.9

He gives estimates of prevalence of these grades in adults in the UK today. These are not much more than informed guesses, but in my view they are sensible. He puts 0.05 per cent of the adult population in Grade III, about four per cent in Grade II and between 25 and 35 per cent in Grade I.

Grade III is fortunately uncommon. These are the real fatties that all of us see occasionally in the street. They are a familiar sight in hospital obesity clinics. With various vigorous treatments most of them can be made to lose weight but in the majority of cases this loss is not maintained. The outlook is very uncertain and their life expectancy is low.

Grade II obesity is a major disease, mainly because it predisposes to high blood pressure and diabetes and is associated with a reduced life expectancy. It is also a contributory factor in the development of many medical disorders. Therefore it requires to be treated seriously. Fortunately treatment can be very successful. In many patients with hypertension or diabetes, the blood pressure or blood glucose becomes normal when the excess of weight is lost, and they are free of symptoms and do not require drugs. Weight loss is seldom easily attained and most patients require detailed professional advice and instruction from dietitians and doctors plus a long period of supervision. Grade II obesity is a major problem for the resources of the health services.

Grade I obesity is not associated with major hazards to health. Actuarial data provided by life insurance companies show that the relationship between life expectation and Quetelet's Index is J-shaped. It has a broad flat optimum between 20 and 28. Mortality is a little higher in very thin people with a lower index. Above 28 mortality rises at first very slowly, but does not begin to rise steeply until values above 32. When the index is between 35 and 40 mortality is from two to three times greater than at the optimum level.

3 Plumpness is not obesity

Men and women with an index between 25 and 30 cannot be said to be suffering from obesity but are properly described as plump. Plump people do not need to reduce their weight for health reasons, though they should watch their weight and see that they do not become obese.

The plump supply by far the greater part of the support for the huge slimming industry – some £200 million on special foods and £2 million on magazines and other literature annually. This is money spent on keeping up with a modern fashion. Any visitor to one of the great galleries of European art who looks at the nudes can see that few of the models used by artists in Renaissance Italy and by painters such as Rembrandt in Flanders were slim. There is no harm in being fashionable, but fashions should not be carried to extremes.

Fashions have their dangers. When I was a medical student in the 1930s anorexia nervosa had a very small space in medical textbooks and we very rarely saw a case. Now it is widely known and there is a large literature on the subject. Always a serious disease and difficult to treat, it carries a significant mortality rate. Most cases start from excessive and unreasonable dietary restrictions aimed at producing a slim figure. It is a high price to pay for trying to keep fashionable.

4 Artificial foods

Totally artificial foods made up of almost chemically pure carbohydrates, fats and proteins with added vitamins and minerals have for many years been available in chemist shops. Even if accurately formulated, they have no nutritional advantage over a diet made up of natural foods. At best they may be useful as a gimmick which may be of temporary help to some people trying to break bad food habits.

An obese patient who is instructed in how to prepare a natural diet providing only 1,000 kcal daily and who is well-motivated and sticks to the instructions should lose one to 1.5 kilogrammes (two–three pounds) a week. It is better for such patients to learn to use natural foods in a manner appropriate for their condition rather than depend on a formula diet. Such patients have no need to spend their money buying a diet from a chemist shop.

An obese patient who wishes to lose 20 kilogrammes of weight can be told that it is realistic to achieve this within 20 weeks, provided they adhere to instructions and that after this time they will be able to increase their food intake sufficiently to sustain their target weight. For the real fatties (Garrow's Grade III obesity) who may have 50–70 kilogrammes of excess fat, it would take one to two years of perseverance with a 1,000 calorie diet before this could be lost. This is a daunting prospect. For such patients a reduction of intake to as low as 300 calories daily will greatly increase the rate of weight loss. This is not without its risks, but for selected patients under medical supervision it can be recommended for periods up to four weeks. There is no way of making 300 calories look like a normal diet. Patients may find it easier to give up all normal foods and to take a liquid formula diet three times a day.

5 The Cambridge diet

There are and have been many formula diets on the market. Of these, the Cambridge diet is perhaps the best known. It has been widely promoted in the USA and three million people there are said to have used it. Promotion is beginning here. A book entitled *The Cambridge Diet* by Alan Howard now has a prominent place on the shelves marked Health in the shops of booksellers. The diet has a legitimate, but small, place in modern medicine. It has been, as case histories in Howard's book relate, the means whereby some patients have lost large amounts of weight (85 kg in 15 months in one case). But such patients could have lost weight similarly on a restricted diet of natural foods. There is no specific indication for the use of an artificial diet. Furthermore these low liquid diets are potentially dangerous. There are known to have been over 150 deaths in the USA among patients on such diets. Most of these have occurred during the use of formulae other than the Cambridge diet and no death can be attributed with certainty to its use. In the UK the Cambridge diet cannot be purchased from chemists' shops but is available from 'controllers' who can be contacted by post. Who those controllers are and the nature and extent of their training is not known to the public. They are not qualified dietitians or doctors. It is now established that disorders of cardiac function may occur in patients who are rapidly losing large amounts of weight and that this is a potentially lethal complication of the prolonged use of restricted diets (T.B. Van Italie & M.U. Yang *American Journal of Clinical Nutrition* Vol. 39, 1984, pp 695–702). All patients on the Cambridge diet or any other low energy diet for a long period should therefore be under close medical supervision, in many cases preferably in hospital.

6 Don't worry about plumpness but treat obesity seriously

The proportion of the body that is fat varies greatly and over a wide range; this does not necessarily affect health. Women on average have about twice as much fat as men and yet are at least as healthy and they live longer. Some of us are naturally lean and remain so throughout life. Others are naturally plump and gain weight easily if they do not curb their appetite. These differences are part of our constitution, to use an old term, and probably determined by our genes. In many societies in the past it has been fashionable to be plump. Today fashion dictates that we should be lean. Fashion is a folly. It leads to simple people losing their money to the smart and unscrupulous. Many millions of pounds and dollars are lost each year this way to the entrepreneurs of the slimming business.

But it would be wrong to end on a note of folly. Obesity is a serious disorder and should be treated seriously. Treatment is always hard and arduous, and usually needs to be lifelong. The necessary dietary restrictions can only be kept up by those who are well motivated and they need expert advice and guidance from the dietetic and medical professions.

9 The Conditions for a Healthy Diet: The 100 Per Cent Unrefined Whole-Truth, Please

Anthony R. Leeds

1 Ground rules for debate

The current debate about diet and health occurring privately and publicly would be more constructive and less acrimonious if the participants accepted the following statements and conditions:

- deciding what to do about diet and health consists of two quite distinct processes: firstly, interpretation of scientific evidence and secondly, deciding what to do as a consequence of what is known
- we should weight the views of debaters according to their background experience and qualifications
- everyone involved in this debate should be consistent within himself so that he would be as reasonable in front of a television camera as when having a discussion with a colleague some hours later
- we should avoid our tendency (probably based on an inbuilt survival feature demanding that all others be classified as friend or foe) to label scientists, health educators or other professionals with simple labels, for example, 'pro-sugar', 'anti-fibre', 'a man with a mission'
- the funding by National Councils of Research of questions relating to nutrition should be adequate and not fall in the void between the Medical Research Council and the Agricultural and Food Research Council; the former seeing nutrition as the responsibility of the latter and *vice versa*
- the professions should not assume that the public cannot understand anything except a simple message.

2 Don't confuse present *policy* decisions with *scientific* conclusions

Interpretation of scientific evidence and deciding what to do, ie, formulation of policy, make quite different intellectual demands on thinkers.

Both are problem-solving, the former demanding that a hypothesis be proved (or resisting attempts to disprove it) and the latter reflecting the general process, occurring in medical practice, where some sort of diagnosis has to be made and a course of management chosen, based on whatever information, however incomplete, is available. We also have to consider the possibility that while some scientists, doctors and health educators are good at both, some may not be, being good at one process only or applying the wrong thinking process to the problem. This may result in a demand for rigorous scientific proof before a policy decision is made or, possibly worse, that inadequate scientific evidence is used to make what is claimed to be a scientific conclusion.

It seems to me to be not unreasonable to make a policy decision in the presence of very little scientific evidence provided that it is clear that it is a 'policy decision' and not a 'scientific conclusion' and provided that the weaknesses of the supporting evidence are stated and the possibilities that the policy may prove to be ineffective or even dangerous are also stated. In practice, the problem for diet and health questions is: how much scientific evidence is needed before a policy decision can be made? This is very much a question of judgement, and in individuals may depend very much on features of personality or even on political belief.

3 Be clear what the experts are experts on

Regarding eligibility for combat, here we have a problem of identity: what is a nutritionist? We have state-registered dietitians, most of whom have a university degree in nutrition. The nation's resource of professional knowledge of nutrition rests very largely with the dietitians. The number of non-dietitian nutritionists with a degree in nutrition is very small. Most of the participants in the debate do not have degrees in nutrition. However, lack of possession of a degree in nutrition need not be a disqualifying feature – relevant experience might be an acceptable substitute.

Another problem related to eligibility is insight into the limits of one's own ability and knowledge. I know from my own experience of teaching many hundreds of university students that this varies enormously. Some cannot see where the limits of their ability lie, while others can. I personally cannot claim to be able to do more than attempt to interpret the scientific evidence and hold some views on the practicalities of implementing dietary change based on my scientific and clinical experience respectively. I know nothing of economic factors in relation to food consumption and very little of the general principles of health education for large groups of people. I am certainly not an investigative journalist, thus you must weight this chapter carefully and accept it in part or, if you wish, dismiss it totally.

Regarding consistency of approach within an individual, while this would be less acceptable to media people, as qualified statements are not very entertaining, I for one would be less perplexed by fellow scientists, who seem perfectly rational when I talk to them but change under stress.

4 Don't exaggerate partisanship

I have worked in the area of dietary fibre for ten years and have been labelled as a 'fibre-man', worse, as a 'bran-man', and people have assumed and have implied that I advocate high-fibre diets. The label has led to a prejudicial judgement about what they think I am. In this case the judgement is wrong. I don't advocate anything in particular, though I think it highly probable that increasing dietary fibre (whatever that is) may be beneficial for some people.

Labels lead to aggression which perhaps even pushes some people to accept their labels (some like to be labelled, some don't). My approach to this problem is to ask: 'Is he really as "anti-sugar" (or "pro-fibre") as he is made out to be?', and when I talk to him he turns out to be perfectly rational – the label had been attached by other people.

5 Don't dismiss research because it is funded by a potentially interested party

Related to the problem of personal labels is the lack of central funding for nutrition research. This drives research workers to seek funding from food producers, manufacturers and distributors (who else is going to pay for it?) so that such workers can have their work dismissed as being suspect because it is funded by a food producer, or can be slandered (usually privately) as being twisters of the truth: 'Of course eating two ounces of rhubarb once a fortnight is good for you, he's funded by the World Rhubarb Organisation's European Office in Brussels – what else do you expect?' Yes, all sponsorship must be stated (this should be a condition of sponsorship) but dismiss the work on technical faults of design, execution or misinterpretation, not on grounds of sponsorship.

6 Don't over-simplify the message to the public

To turn now to simple messages: apart from reflecting arrogance, simple messages cause much friction among professionals. A simple message (in this field) is an incomplete message. However, there are consumer surveys which show that quite large numbers of people don't understand even basic nutritional terms and there are those who argue that since only 30 per cent of the population will understand a complex message, a simple message should be given to all. Once again the mass approach. Yet these same people want to give messages about heart disease to the 70 per cent who will not die from it, as well as the 30 per cent or so who will.

Why can't the general principle of giving to everyone that which will only be of benefit to one in three apply to the complexity of the message as well as to its content? The 30 per cent who receive the message may pass it on to the other 70 per cent better than we can. I would prefer to be guilty of causing confusion rather than of talking-down to people. Much argument occurs because of a view that a simple message is incomplete and to some extent dishonest.

7 Distinguish between the needs of individuals and those of populations

While it is a perfectly reasonable approach to advise populations as a whole to make dietary changes, at the final site of battle (the 'fridge door, the polystyrene carton, or the dinner plate) food is eaten by individuals who have individual needs: the needs of children for normal growth and development, the needs of pregnancy and lactation, the needs of the elderly with increasingly inefficient absorptive systems and demineralising skeletons. The special requirements of sub-groups of the population and of individuals within these sub-groups have perhaps not been considered as fully as they might. It is also often forgotten that food contains nutrients other than those half a dozen or so implicated in the degenerative diseases of Western civilisation: nutrients such as iron and calcium which may be needed in greater quantity by some than by others. Have we really considered all of the *nutritional* implications of some of the changes we advocate?

If I may quote two anecdotal examples: there are verbal case reports of children with growth failure as a consequence of high fibre diets (so bulky that insufficient energy is eaten); and I have seen iron deficiency anaemia in older women almost certainly exacerbated by low-fat diets which also happen to be low in iron. Both of these situations are fairly predictable and underline the need for individual guidance on dietary change.

8 Present the whole dietary truth

Another major argument concerns the problem of identifying individuals at risk of degenerative disease in whom preventive action may be beneficial. If the specificity of tests was high and costs low, no doubt this approach would have been chosen. With the development of new and better blood tests, as will certainly occur, the need for dietary change in entire populations may diminish. In the meantime, population change for specific purposes is judged as being the right policy. Public education is required to achieve the objectives, but I would appeal for a presentation of the whole story with all its qualifications and uncertainties so that, should a change of direction become necessary, the experts will not have got it wrong again.

10 Diet and Disease: Nonsense and Non-science

James Le Fanu

1 Contradictions in dietary advice

Over the last 50 years, nutritionists have generated two completely contradictory sets of recommendations as to what constitutes a 'healthy diet'. From the 1930s onwards people were encouraged to consume dairy products especially milk, eggs, butter and meat in place of 'poor quality' foods such as bread and potatoes. Over the last five years this advice has been reversed and people are now advised to cut down on their intake of dairy foods by as much as one third and increase consumption of bread, cereals and pasta. This chapter attempts to provide explanations for this interesting nonsense.

Both sets of recommendations are, in their own way, plausible. In the depressed years of the 1930s it was appropriate to suggest that the 'physique of the nation' was imperilled by chronic malnourishment (which could be corrected by increasing intake of dairy foods); and in the 1970s it seemed obvious that heart disease was a disease of over-consumption (which could be prevented by reducing intake of dairy foods). But it is necessary to look behind the powerful imagery both of the characterisation of the problems and of their proffered solutions. Indeed, food itself is so run through with sexual and class-based connotations that it is mandatory to evaluate critically the scientific credentials of the contending arguments.

An obvious possibility is that there has been some recent revolutionary discovery in nutritional science itself which has led to the overthrow of the old orthodoxy; but this is transparently not the case. The scientific basis of nutrition, the concept of energy balance, the discovery of the essential vitamins and minerals was all basically achieved by the 1930s. If anything, it can be said we 'know' less about 'good' nutrition now than we did then, as more has been revealed about the variability and adaptability of the human organism to different dietary patterns.

So to find the requisite explanations it is necessary to look elsewhere, to *theories* of what constitutes a 'healthy' diet and the psychological and political determinants of those theories. It will be seen that the justification of both sets of dietary recommendations relies on partial and selective interpretation of the facts; that their wide adoption reflects the success of self-interested sections of the scientific community in providing messages that mirror society's views of itself. Armed with a historical perspective of the changing fashions of nutritional advice, it is then possible to assess the harm of current nutritional enthusiasms.

2 The basic rules – enough food, not too much, and a balanced diet

It is appropriate to start with a nutritional truism whose importance is that it is significantly absent from any discussion about 'healthy diets': societies have prospered, and prosper now, with a virtually infinite variety of patterns of food consumption. From the Kalahari Desert to the Alaskan wastes, from the Indian plains to New York City people live, work, reproduce and sustain their cultures whether their diet consists of 1,500 or 3,500 calories per day, whether those calories come from predominantly animal or vegetable sources, or a broad mix of the two. This facility, that far outstretches that of any other mammals, can be attributed to two important features of human society: that man is an omnivore and so (unlike the panda doomed for ever to patrol the bamboo forests of Northern China) can find nourishment from a wide variety of food sources; and that man is intelligent and so can transform those food sources into edible products, most obviously by cooking.

There are two constraints on this adaptability. Inadequate amounts of food or overconsumption will lead to malnutrition and obesity respectively. And a severely unbalanced diet can lead to specific vitamin or mineral deficiences that can be corrected by adding the missing elements to the diet.

3 Dietary advice infected with partisan theories

If man can survive, granted an adequate source of food energy with a wide variety of diets, then the advocacy of first a high dairy intake and then a low dairy intake as the basis of a 'healthy diet' is likely to rely on partisan theories of good nutrition. This is indeed the case. The promotion of increased dairy food consumption in the 1930s relied on the concept of man fulfilling his 'genetic potential'. Consider two groups of boys in the 1930s attending, say, a secondary school in Bermondsey and Eton. In nutritional terms they can be distinguished because whereas the diet of the Etonians is rich and diverse, that of the Bermondsey bruisers is filling and monotonous. Both groups are healthy in that they have no stigmata of specific nutritional deficiency, they are active, run around and misbehave as children tend to do. However, the average height of the Etonians is an inch or two more than that of the Bermondseyites. There is probably a partial genetic explanation for this, but if the Bermondsey boys were fed the Etonian diet they might grow faster and so end up taller than they would otherwise have been (that is, they would have fulfilled their 'genetic potential') but they do not *need* the Etonian diet in order to be healthy because they have *adapted* to their own diet.

If nutritional health is defined in functional terms both groups of children are equal. But if nutritional health is defined as the ability of all children to grow to the height of the Etonians, then one could say the Bermondsey boys are 'chronically malnourished'. And it is this idea of 'chronic malnourishment' that allowed the British nutritionist, John Boyd Orr, to argue in the 1930s that more than 50 per cent of the population were eating an inadequate diet and that to achieve optimal nutritional health there needed to be a major increase in what he described as 'protective foods', especially milk, butter, meat, eggs and vegetables.

In practical terms he defined optimal nutrition as that enjoyed by his own class and 'chronic malnourishment' as anything less than this. His nutritional recommendations were strongly based on a eugenic concept of a 'healthy nation' (ie, that everyone should have the physical characteristics of the upper class).

4 Current dietary advice based on misinterpreting cross-cultural studies

By contrast, the theoretical basis for the current set of nutritional recommendations for a *reduced* consumption of dairy foods comes from a completely different source, outside the strict confines of nutritional science. The Diet-Disease hypothesis, as it will be called, derives its major scientific authority from *cross cultural* studies where the patterns of food intake and disease in different countries are compared. Salt intake correlates with the incidence of hypertension, fat intake with heart disease and cancers, fibre intake with bowel cancer and appendicitis, and so on.

The first and most important point is that these correlations do not necessarily indicate a causal relationship. The countries under comparison vary far more widely than just in the types of food they consume. The correlation of fat consumption and breast cancer in Figure 1 illustrates the pitfalls. Looked at simplistically one could argue (as do the Diet-disease protagonists) that the graph proves that fat intake *causes* breast cancer. But we know a few more things about the natural history of

Figure 1.

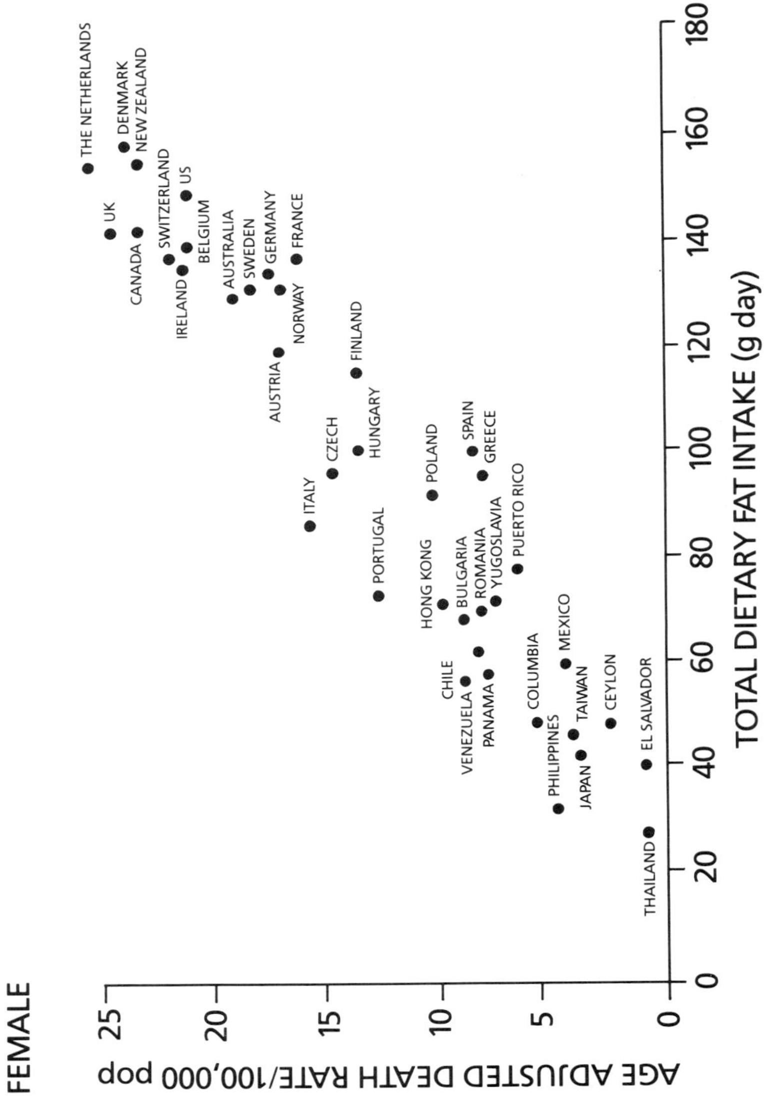
FEMALE
AGE ADJUSTED DEATH RATE/100,000 pop
0
5
10
15
20
25
TOTAL DIETARY FAT INTAKE (g day)
0
20
40
60
80
100
120
140
160
180
THE NETHERLANDS
DENMARK
NEW ZEALAND
UK
CANADA
SWITZERLAND
US
IRELAND
BELGIUM
AUSTRALIA
SWEDEN
GERMANY
NORWAY
FRANCE
AUSTRIA
FINLAND
CZECH
HUNGARY
ITALY
POLAND
SPAIN
GREECE
PORTUGAL
HONG KONG
BULGARIA
ROMANIA
YUGOSLAVIA
PUERTO RICO
CHILE
VENEZUELA
PANAMA
COLUMBIA
MEXICO
PHILIPPINES
TAIWAN
JAPAN
CEYLON
EL SALVADOR
THAILAND

breast cancer that permit a different interpretation. Firstly, that the risk of breast cancer increases the earlier that menstruation starts (and menstruation starts earlier in developed countries). Secondly, that the risk increases the longer that the first pregnancy is delayed (another feature of developed countries). So all this graph is showing is that breast cancer increases with the 'development' of a society, and more developed societies have a higher fat consumption. The correlation though suggesting a *causal* relationship in fact is only reflecting an *associative* one.

5 Tougher tests before conclusions

The founding fathers of epidemiology were only too aware of the dangers of confusing *cause* with *association* and so established certain 'tests' which a correlation had to pass if it was to be genuinely considered as indicating a causal relationship. Does the correlation hold within countries as well as between countries? Is there a dose-response relationship, eg, do higher rates of fat intake predictably increase the risk of heart disease? Does the correlation hold over time, eg, are changing patterns of heart disease reflected in changing patterns of food consumption? What is the effect of testing the correlation, eg, if people are encouraged to reduce their fat intake does this reduce the risk of heart disease? And so on. These are the epidemiological equivalents to Koch's postulates for proving that an organism really does cause the disease with which it is found in association. They are critical, for no matter how interesting the cross-cultural observations might be, if the hypotheses they generate are not confirmed by the above tests, the link between diet and disease falls down. This leaves two possible conclusions: first, we do not know why there are major differences in disease patterns between different countries; and secondly, diet is not a modifiable cause of heart disease, hypertension, cancers, etc. It so happens that the hypotheses generated by the cross-cultural studies are *not* sustained by critical testing. One interesting part of the diet-disease story is how its protagonists have attempted to deny this.

Finally, it is important to note that medicine's strength has always been empiricism rather than an understanding of the basic mechanisms of disease. So we know that we can treat diabetes with insulin but we do not know the cause of diabetes. Indeed apart from infectious and genetic diseases it is only possible to attribute a cause to about one per cent of the diseases in the medical textbook (smoking and lung disease is an example). So when an all-embracing theory arrives on the scene to argue that 'small beneficial changes in diet' will prevent diseases as complex as heart disease, hypertension and cancer it is likely to be fraudulent.

6 The temptation to go beyond the evidence

London: November 2nd, 1936

> In a downpour of rain on Saturday afternoon the Jarrow unemployed marchers made their way into London still stepping out briskly and cheerfully as they completed the last stage of their 300 mile journey on foot...the men were frequently greeted with shouts of "Good Luck", and from North Country people who had turned out to greet them "Good old Tyneside"...all but four of them have been continuously treated for blistered feet on the march, but none of them would drop out for this reason...

In the House of Commons at the time the Jarrow marchers were 'stepping out' on the first stage of their epic march to London, Mr. Tim Johnston for the Labour opposition 'brought forward a motion declaring that the House noted with concern the convincing evidence of widespread malnutrition'. Amongst the evidence he cited was the recent study *Family, Health and Income*, from Sir John Boyd Orr which had shown that 'four and a half million people were endeavouring to live at a standard below the minimum and that their diet was deficient in every constituent'. Boyd Orr had also shown that there were a further nine million people whose diet was defective in 'protective constituents'. Johnston proceeded to crucify the Government for allowing a situation where 'side by side with want and malnourishment, there was organised limitation of production and restriction of the market'.

It is difficult to underestimate the significance of this particular congruence of political interest and scientific authority. The malnourishment issue was to become a stick with which the Labour opposition was to attack the Government on many occasions in the coming years: it moved nutrition into the central stage of the political arena and catapulted Boyd Orr to fame as a national figure – the scientist who dared to tell the truth. But what *was* the evidence for widespread chronic malnourishment?

Family, Health and Income had investigated the diet of 1,350 families stratified into six classes according to their average expenditure on food. Perhaps not surprisingly, it had shown marked differences. The amounts of bread and flour consumed per person were roughly the same, but animal fat, vegetables, fruit and fish rose steadily up through the classes. Boyd Orr then compared the dietary intakes of calcium, vitamin A, iron and phosphorus in the different classes with the amounts 'required for health' as laid down by the US Government Bureau of Home Economics and concluded that 'a diet completely adequate for health according to modern standards is reached at an income level above that of half the population'. Therefore 50 per cent of the population were 'chronically malnourished'.

However, Boyd Orr had been unable to turn up any evidence of widespread clinical malnutrition in his study. Anaemia, chronic infection of the upper respiratory tract, skeletal deformities typical of rickets and tooth decay were all rare and not found significantly more in the lower social classes. A 'feeding experiment' in which some children had their diets supplemented by dairy foods also failed to show benefit in terms of more rapid growth. So he was left with the comparative differences in height between children of different social classes as evidence for his thesis. The boys at Christ's Hospital public school, he noted, were at the age of 17 'on average three inches taller than employed males of the same age'.

This does not mean however, that there was not chronic ill health in the 1930s. The lethal childhood infections, tuberculosis, valvular heart disease secondary to rheumatic fever were all much more common than now, and more prevalent in the lower social classes. Further it was the opinion of some medical officers that children *did* appear malnourished, though their subjective observations were difficult to replicate. Nonetheless Boyd Orr's thesis that *50 per cent* of the population were malnourished went way beyond what could legitimately be inferred from his study.

It is easy with hindsight to see the source of his erroneous conclusions. He was working at the exciting time of the discovery of vitamins and it was tempting to over-interpret the new knowledge. If gross vitamin deficiency led to clinically definable medical conditions, then perhaps 'minor' vitamin deficiencies might be a cause of chronic ill health. The figures of recommended dietary intakes of nutrients that he used as a comparison for the diets of the lower social classes were arbitrary, and so the implication that people consuming less were at a disadvantage was not justifiable. His own definition of 'optimal nutritional health' as 'a state of health such that no improvement could be effected by diet' was in scientific terms impossible to prove. And finally the characterisation of dairy foods as being 'better' than others stemmed primarily from a psychological association of these foods with upper class patterns of consumption.

Two classical experiments in the succeeding years, one 'natural' the other man-made, finally refuted his thesis of the nutritional need to increase consumption of dairy foods. The 'natural' experiment was the Second World War in which rationing imposed on the British people a diet that bore a striking resemblance to that which had 'caused' chronic malnourishment amongst the lower social classes. It was high in carbohydrates, cereals and vegetables, low in 'protective' dairy foods as Table 1 shows. Nursing mothers and infants received special allowances

Table 1: Average adult ration per week

Bacon and ham	4 oz (100g)
Meat	to the value of 1s. 2d. (6p today). Sausages were not rationed but difficult to obtain; offal was originally unrationed but sometimes formed part of the meat ration.
Butter	2 oz (50 g)
Cheese	2 oz (50 g) sometimes it rose to 4 oz (100 g) and even up to 8 oz (225 g)
Margarine	4 oz (100 g)
Cooking fat	4 oz (100 g) often dropping to 2 oz (50 g)
Milk	3 pints (1800 ml) sometimes dropping to 2 pints (1200 ml.) Household (skimmed dried) milk was available, I think this was 1 packet each 4 weeks.
Sugar	8 oz (225 g)
Preserves	1 lb (450 g) every 2 months
Tea	2 oz (50 g)
Eggs	1 shell egg a week if available but at times dropping to 1 every two weeks. Dried eggs – 1 packet each 4 weeks.
Sweets	12 oz (350 g) each 4 weeks.

of milk and bread was fortified with calcium. By the simple criteria of infant and maternal mortality, the health of the nation improved and there was a general feeling that people were 'healthier' (though they found the dietary restrictions onerous) and all this was achieved without the major increases in 'protective foods' advocated by Boyd Orr.

The man-made experiment was conducted in German orphanages in the aftermath of the war by McCance and Widdowson under the auspices of the Medical Research Council. They had set out to resolve another longstanding nutritional conundrum – whether brown bread was more nutritious than white. The children had had little to eat for some time and were obviously undernourished, weighing 10 per cent less than American children of the same age. They were allocated extra supplements of either white or brown bread and were in fact receiving 75 per cent of their total calories from this source, along with 80 mls. of milk per day and a small amount of animal protein. Both groups of children rapidly put on weight but interestingly there was no difference between the two groups. With such a high proportion of bread in the diet and so little 'protective' food it was expected that the differing nutritional qualities of the two types of bread would become apparent but it did not. In a further study, two groups of children were given the same amount of bread but one group was given an extra supplement of 500 mls. of milk per day. Again both groups of children grew satisfactorily and there was no difference between the two groups.

McCance and Widdowson concluded:

> This was a most valuable experiment because it showed what good food bread could be for growing children when the rest of the diet contained very little milk, animal protein and other 'protective foods'...that wheat flour had a nutritive value for growing children far beyond that usually assigned to it in recent years.

Neither of these experiments seemed to influence people's conception of what constituted a 'healthy diet' in the succeeding decades. The powerful imagery that Boyd Orr had evoked of whole classes suffering from chronic ill health because their diet was deficient in 'protective' dairy foods persisted.

7 Nutritionists meddling in politics

One can be charitable towards Boyd Orr and argue that at least his polemic on behalf of dairy foods ensured the promotion and extension of free milk for schoolchildren and the school dinner service. But 'bad science makes worse social policy' and if his arguments did little harm in Britain they probably vitiated the programmes against world malnutrition that were set up after the War. At the end of the War Boyd Orr became the first Director of the Food and Agricultural Organisation (FAO) where he promoted an erroneous and harmful understanding of the extent of world hunger and what its solution might be. Again his arbitrary definition of malnutrition grossly exaggerated the extent of the problem, thus blunting the response of the relevant agencies. Once more the issue was simplistically reduced to a single problem except this time it was 'the protein gap' rather than lack of 'protective foods' and enormous energies were directed towards filling 'the gap' until the concept was refuted in the 1970s. Only recently has it become acceptable to acknowledge that malnutrition is a complex issue which stretches well beyond the simple question of inadequate food supplies. Only by defining it accurately is it possible to find a solution, a process that Boyd Orr may well have hindered for a couple of decades.

8 NACNE – going beyond the evidence again

In 1983 the NACNE Report was published in an atmosphere of considerable recrimination. The powerful food lobby, it was alleged, had attempted to suppress the Report's important 'findings' about the close relationship between diet and disease. Among other things, the Report asserted that the epidemic of heart disease was due to the nation's fondness for dairy foods; strokes were caused by an addiction to salt; obesity and dental caries were due to excess sugar consumption; and cancer of the colon, appendicitis and other gastro/intestinal diseases were caused by an inadequate intake of fibre in the form of bread and cereals. The Report then made major recommendations: dairy foods should be reduced by one third; salt and sugar consumption halved; and there should be a major increase in the consumption of bread and pasta. It was high noon for the traditional British way of cooking for though the finger might have pointed at specific foods it was actually incriminating a cultural way of life – bacon and eggs, fish and chips, cakes and puddings. The 'healthy diet' of the previous four decades had been reversed, with a vengeance.

It was taken up with enthusiasm by 'community dietitians' and 'health educators'. For example, children are now taught, *inter alia*, that fish and chips cause heart disease and that they should not eat crisps and nuts because their added salt is 'harmful'. The media has revelled in the story of wicked food companies and corrupt doctors wheeling and dealing to suppress this crucial information that could prevent 'tens of thousands of premature deaths' each year.

However the evidence in favour of these radical reductions in dairy food consumption is no better than Boyd Orr was able to provide for his thesis of chronic malnourishment preventable by *increasing* dairy food consumption. The diet-heart hypothesis will be considered in most detail.

9 Fat and heart disease – the thesis which leaks like a collander

From the mid-1920s in the US and the UK and, subsequently, in other countries, doctors began to notice an alarming increase in deaths from heart disease amongst middle-aged men. Rapidly and inexorably the toll rose so that by the 1950s it had become the commonest cause of premature male death – and still it kept rising. The explanation was by no means clear but it was felt the problem was probably related to an abnormality in the circulation of the blood in the arteries leading to the heart. For the first 15 years after the war the leading theory was that it was a clotting abnormality, but for a variety of reasons this theory fell into disfavour. Attention then turned to the lining of the arteries and in particular the accretion of cholesterol-rich plaques (atheroma) that interrupted the flow of blood. It was postulated that the amount of atheroma was influenced by the consumption of dairy foods high in saturated fat.

The most direct evidence in favour of this theory was the famous *Cross-cultural* study initiated by Ancel Keys in which he compared the incidence of heart disease in selected groups in different countries (eg USA and Japan) and showed a correlation with the consumption of dairy foods. Later it was shown that when Japanese migrants moved to the US their risk of heart disease increased – a phenomenon attributed to a change in diet. Laboratory studies showed that varying the types of fat in the diet could influence the level of cholesterol in the blood. The famous Framingham study in the US showed there was an increased risk of heart disease in individuals with very high blood cholesterol levels. And so the diet-heart disease was born. Saturated fat in the diet increases the cholesterol in the blood that increases the amount of atheroma in the arteries that has led to the epidemic of heart disease.

Certainly this thesis is plausible, but it leaks like a collander. Each supposition sustaining it is run through with contradictions. First, a series of autopsy studies performed at a time of rapidly increasing heart disease *failed* to show a parallel increase in the amount or severity of atheroma. Secondly, the cross-cultural correlation of fat intake and heart disease does *not* hold when similar countries are being compared (see Figure 2). In addition, within one country the risk of heart disease is *not* related to the amount of fat in the diet. Thirdly, the migrant studies do *not* show that a change in diet increases the risk of heart disease since it is a generalised and unexplained phenomenon that migrant communities

Figure 2: Coronary mortality and total fat intake in various countries.

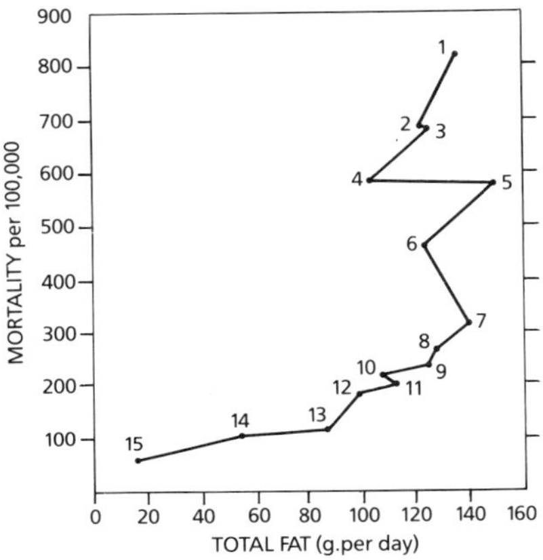

Mortality refers to number of men aged 55–64 in 100,000 certified as dying of coronary disease in 1952. The numbers refer to countries in order of decreasing mortality as follows: (1) U.S.A., (2) Australia, (3) Canada, (4) Finland, (5) New Zealand, (6) United Kingdom, (7) Denmark, (8) Sweden, (9) Norway, (10) Netherlands, (11) Switzerland, (12) Western Germany, (13) France, (14) Italy, (15) Japan.

acquire the pattern of disease of their adopted countries. Fourthly, it is *very difficult* to manipulate the level of cholesterol in the blood by changing the types of fat in the diet because the cholesterol level is itself under the control of powerful homeostatic mechanisms in the body that ensure it remains within tightly-controlled limits. Finally, the increased risk of heart disease in those with a high cholesterol level is not because they eat more dairy foods than anyone else, but because they have a biochemical abnormality of fat transport in the body.

It is therefore possible to rewrite the diet-heart hypothesis. Fat consumption has a minimal effect on blood cholesterol. Most people with heart disease have a normal cholesterol level. There are however a group of people with increased risk of the disease, but their high cholesterol level is not related to the amount of fat in their diet. The fundamental cause of heart disease is not known, a high cholesterol level is merely an additional, not a determinant cause of the disease.

10 The verdict of experiment – fat reduction does not significantly reduce heart disease

To resolve the dispute between the diet-heart hypothesis and the non-diet-heart hypothesis it is necessary to appeal to the arbitration court of science – the experiment. This alone will indicate which of the two hypotheses is correct. There are two ways of experimentally testing the hypotheses. First, by encouraging a group of people to change their diet and see if this reduces the incidence of heart disease. If it does, the diet-heart hypothesis stands. But if it only does so in those with very high cholesterol levels, the non-diet-heart disease hypothesis is confirmed. Secondly, by examining the changing pattern of heart disease to see if it is reflected in radical changes in dietary patterns. If it is not, then again the diet-heart disease hypothesis falls.

It is possible to submit the hypothesis to both these tests and so confident were the protagonists of the diet-heart hypothesis that (unwisely as it turned out) they set about testing it in the largest and most expensive set of trials in the history of medicine. In Europe and the USA middle-aged men were recruited in vast numbers – 60,000 in all – for massive control trials in which one half were encouraged to reduce their fat consumption, stop smoking and be treated for high blood pressure if necessary. These were the 'intervention' group. The remaining 30,000 acted as controls.

There were four important trials: MRFIT and WHO in men with normal cholesterol levels and the OSLO and LRCCPPT trial in men with abnormally high levels of cholesterol in the blood. All that was necessary then was to sit back and wait for the results to roll in showing the efficacy of recommending low fat diets. The results were certainly impressive in their consistency. In the MRFIT and WHO trials, the recommendations to reduce fat consumption had *no* effect on either mortality from heart disease or on total mortality.

In the OSLO and LRCCPPT trial the risk of heart disease *was* reduced in the intervention group, but only down to the level of the rest of the population and there was *no* difference in total mortality. The famous Karelia study in Finland came to similar conclusions. This community-based attempt to influence the incidence of heart disease by encouraging people to adopt a low fat diet is claimed as evidence for the diet-heart disease hypothesis. Unfortunately, although heart disease did fall during the period of the study it was also, for unknown reasons, falling throughout Finland at the same time. So by the end of the project Karelia still had the highest rate of heart disease in the country and the decline was no greater than that in a 'control' province, Kuopio.

The second test of the hypothesis is to compare the changing patterns of heart disease in different countries with changing patterns of food consumption. Since 1968 there has been a markedly precipitate decline in heart disease in several countries simultaneously; the mirror image of the rise that occurred in the 1930s and 1940s. This decline is most marked in Australia, New Zealand, Canada, USA and Japan. It is apparent that

Figure 3: Coronary heart death mortality rates – 100,000 males aged 45–64 compared with trends in fat consumption for USA, Australia, New Zealand, Canada and Japan.

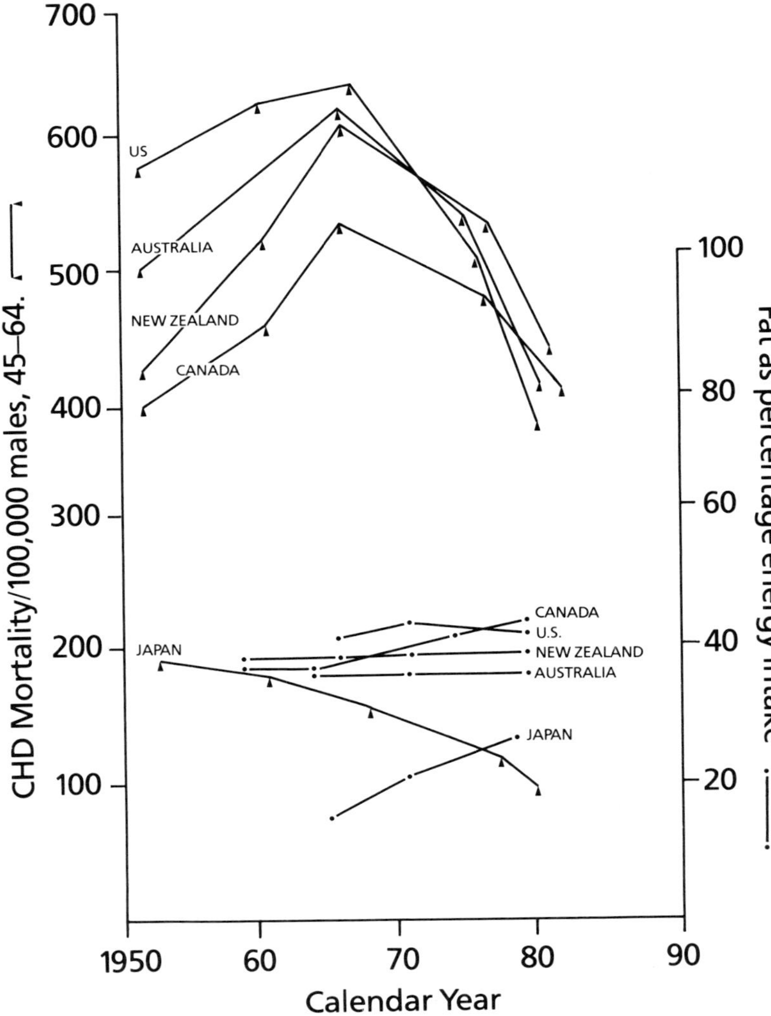

a similar decline is beginning in Britain. But in none of these countries has the decline been parallelled by a radical change in fat consumption as can be seen from Figure 3.

So what conclusions can we draw? It is apparent that if one can identify the small group of people in whom a biochemical abnormality leads to a raised level of cholesterol in the blood, and if one can reduce that level, then their risk of heart disease will fall. This is the 'high risk' strategy for prevention of heart disease. However, for the vast majority of the population diet is not a cause of heart disease and dietary change is ineffective in preventing it. The non-diet-heart hypothesis is upheld.

11 Using propaganda to sell dietary solutions which science won't buy

Rational observers might be hammering the nails into the coffin of the diet-heart hypothesis but its protagonists are reluctant to let go. And why should they since they have the ball and intend to run with it? After 20 years of trying to prove that heart disease is preventable by dietary change, even the most scientifically rigorous might be excused for refusing to accept that their life's work has been spent in pursuit of a chimera. Anyway there are no free airline tickets for those who say the cause of heart disease is not known.

So the last three years have been spent selling the hypothesis in the marketplace. The goods might be shoddy but luckily the public have a touching faith in 'experts'! Two tactics have been adopted. The first is to use expert committees to assert what the scientific evidence so abysmally fails to confirm. There have been a rash of such committees over the last few years – WHO (1982), NACNE (1983), COMA (1984), JACNE (1985). Each has apparently examined the entrails of the evidence and come to the unanimous conclusion that heart disease can after all be prevented if the nation were only to eat a better, 'healthier' diet. If it is that obvious, why the need for all these expert committees, or is the public being sold opinions? The 'experts' certainly have an eclectic attitude to the evidence. None of their reports, for example, point out that the pattern of heart disease is not reflected in changing patterns of food consumption. Three of the four even manage to avoid mentioning the trials.

The second tactic has been to obviate the need for scientific discussion by turning the campaign against heart disease into a national crusade by 'mobilising' the media. The argument goes something like this: the British nation are a greedy and degenerate lot whose fondness for dairy foods, salt and sugar makes them vulnerable to 'killer' diseases such as heart disease (shot here of ambulance screeching through the night). There is 'overwhelming evidence' that if everyone just ate a healthier diet these diseases would be prevented. Mind you the 'evidence' 'does fall short of proof', but we can't wait, we need 'action' now. There are some who dare to challenge the need for 'action now' but they are either lackeys of the food industry or 'not interested in prevention'.

Even though Boyd Orr and the NACNE Report come to such diverse conclusions as to what really constitutes a 'healthy diet', there are striking similarities in their mode of action. Both exploit a politicised view of society, whether it be the 'hungry thirties' or the 'affluent (and greedy) eighties'. Both present an inaccurate view of the health problems of those societies and promote 'better nutrition' as a panacea. Both rely on the over-interpretation of slender theories to justify their position and have a blind spot for any contradictory evidence. Both rely heavily on expert committees to assert what the scientific evidence cannot maintain. Both characterise opposition to their theories as being narrow and reactionary.

But it is difficult to extend the charitable verdict on Boyd Orr's work (he did after all ensure that some children obtained a nutritious food they would not otherwise have received) to the current generation of NACNE-ites. In all their self-righteous admonitions to the public they appear blind to the serious consequences of their propaganda, that it misinforms the public about the complexity of disease, trivialises tragedy, blames patients for their illnesses, stigmatises the dairy industry and degrades medicine as a science-b[illegible]sion.

11 Food Advertising Not the Problem

Charles Plouviez

1 Why health educators distrust advertising

'Go and see what young Johnny is doing and tell him to stop', said the harassed mother in the old story, and her attitude is not unlike that of many health education people to advertising. One obvious reason for this is pragmatic: a ban or restriction on advertising is an extremely public mark of the success of a campaign, even if it makes no real contribution towards achieving that campaign's aims.

But there are more serious reasons why propagandists for health see advertising as a suitable case for treatment, and in this paper I want to examine three of them: firstly an inflated notion of the potency of advertising, often coupled with disappointment about its results in their own sphere; secondly, the authoritarian nature of the medical model, and its unconscious application to matters of health education; and thirdly, a failure to understand the political and social consequences of restrictive legislation in a democratic society.

Advertising people have largely themselves to blame for misunderstandings about the nature of their business. They are notoriously not among the most modest of professionals, they believe – with some cause – that in order to bolster their claim to sell other people's wares they must cry their own wares as loudly as possible, and in consequence they have been guilty of overclaiming for the effects of advertising for the best part of a century. Not surprisingly, their critics, and many neutral bystanders, have chosen to take them at their word, aided by the fact that the evidence for successful advertising campaigns grows apace, while the evidence for failures is too often buried in the archives of advertising agencies and the memories of practitioners.

2 Advertising for preventive health proves not to be a 'magic pill'

Nevertheless, an increasing number of people in the health education field have learned some part of the truth in recent years as a result of their efforts to harness advertising to 'good' causes – to reduce smoking and drinking, prevent accidents, promote contraception, or modify dietary habits. Unfortunately, their failure to achieve the magic results they had expected has often given them a redoubled sense of grievance. Like all unsuccessful advertisers, they simultaneously demand more funds for their campaign, cast doubts on the effectiveness of advertising as a whole, and bewail the fact that what they see as the opposition is, quite unfairly of course, doing better than they are. More than anything else, this paranoid reaction demonstrates a mistaken idea about the nature and limitations of advertising. An important paper presented to the international conference on Health Education and the Media at Edinburgh in March 1981 by B.K. Tones, himself a prominent health educationist and director of the Leeds Diploma course in Health Education puts it succinctly: 'the power of mass media tends to be overemphasised in Health Education – largely due to inappropriate comparisons being made with commercial advertising which usually has lower aspirations and involves fundamentally different processes'.[1]

3 The function of Manufacturers' Consumer Advertising

The most commonly encountered form of commercial advertising is that which is intended to launch or increase the market share of a specific brand of product or service in a marketplace in which other competing brands already exist. This is defined by the industry as Manufacturers' Consumer Advertising (MCA), and although it is only one of a number of methods of achieving this limited end, experience and research studies have both proved that for most mass-produced products in markets where repeat purchasing is frequent it is the most cost-effective.

However, to those not engaged in marketing, the actual results achieved have a puny look. Since the introduction of the Effectiveness Awards scheme by the Institute of Practitioners in Advertising some six years ago, a mass of case history material[2] has been made available which is as near to being scientifically assessable as anything in the human sciences can be, and as well as proving beyond doubt that advertising is cost-effective in promoting brands it shows up the limitations of that effectiveness more clearly than most previous evidence.

For instance, the winner of the Grand Prix in the 1984 Awards was Dulux Natural Whites, a new range of household paints from the country's leading paint manufacturer. After two years and an advertising expenditure close to three million pounds, the brand achieved a market share of 17 per cent of domestic paint sales by volume. As a commercial exercise for ICI, it was a huge success – but it was hardly the kind of magic that advertising's critics tend to attribute to its powers. A total market share of 17 per cent would not, for instance, get far in the direction of returning an Alliance government.

Most advertising campaigns have even more modest aims and achievements to boast of. The case study for St. Ivel Gold, a yellow low-fat spread which under current regulations cannot be described as either butter or margarine but competes with both, reports an expenditure of £5.3 million on TV advertising over three years to achieve a brand share increase from three to six per cent – less than the discrepancy between the ratings of our main political parties as reported most weeks by competing opinion polls.

Almost all the advertising threatened by the health lobby falls into the MCA category, and most of it happens in markets which are 'mature', ie in which little or no total market growth is occurring. The yellow fats market, for instance, has been virtually static for the past decade, the only major changes being, first the swing from butter to margarine in 1975–80, and then the growth of the low-fat sector in the past five years.

Similarly mature or declining markets exist in the UK for confectionery, milk, sugar and many other commodities, so that in these markets the only opportunity a producer has of maintaining or increasing his share of the market is at the expense of his competitors. And this can only be achieved by product development, producing a brand which is in some discernible way better, cheaper, or more consonant with current consumer tastes. This is already leading to important shifts in advertising towards those products which can claim to improve health in the context of the interest stimulated by the NACNE and COMA reports.

The best-researched of the maturer markets throughout the world is that for alcohol. Work done in recent years by the Advertising Association[3] has established, for all but those who cannot believe evidence which conflicts with their prejudices, the futility of attempting to solve the problem of alcohol abuse by banning alcohol advertising. In reviewing a large body of research from all over the world, most of it from non-industry sources, the Advertising Association concludes that it 'clearly suggests that advertising has little or no impact on mature alcohol markets, other than at the brand level'.

The most remarkable demonstration of this comes from France, where the advertising of whisky has been banned since 1957. In that year, whisky imports were 157,000 proof gallons: by 1979 they totalled 6,294,000 proof gallons. Even more alarming was a report by *The Times* Moscow correspondent in 1981 which said 'In spite of an unrelenting campaign against alcohol, stricter laws on the sale of drink, daily temperence propaganda in the press, at school and on the factory floor, the Russians appear powerless against the waves of vodka and wine now washing over the country'.[4]

4 The difficulties of 'advocacy advertising'

Just as advertising can rarely increase or reduce the total size of mature markets, equally it is not by any means the most effective way of changing deeply held prejudices or beliefs among consumers. So-called 'advocacy advertising' has had a chequered career, partly because it has never attracted investment on anything like the scale of brand advertising, but mostly because the research results to date have tended to be ambiguous or discouraging.

This is not surprising. Advertising is at its most effective when it encourages a very large number of people to make a very small change in their behaviour. The choice of a brand of lager is a small thing compared with the decision to wear a seat belt. For many years, advertising campaigns were run by the Central Office of Information (COI) to encourage seat-belt use. The campaigns were carefully measured, and were successful in advertising terms, though never cost-effective. Broadly, when a campaign was running, seat-belt usage rose to around 30 per cent of motorists, only to drop each time the campaign ended to a figure of not much over ten per cent. Advertising on the scale required to get even a bare majority of drivers using belts all the time was out of the question. Advertising would clearly never solve the problem by itself.

Nevertheless, the very fact that the campaigns had run, it is now believed, greatly helped to reinforce the other channels of communication by which public opinion was won over to the idea that seat-belt wearing was a legitimate target of public policy. Legislation could be introduced with virtually none of the opposition which it would have attracted a few years earlier.

Current opinion is that advertising will give saliency to an issue, rather than change attitudes. Most of the people most of the time do not feel strongly on most of the topics of the day; however, if there is an underlying tow of sympathy towards an idea, advertising can put that idea more firmly on the agenda. A clear instance of this occurred in the GLC campaign against its own abolition: it successfully awakened dormant public opinion in favour of a local authority for London, in spite of the initial low popularity of the particular regime led by Ken Livingstone.

5 Why the authoritarian model fails in preventive medicine

Such cumbersome methods of achieving social change do not appeal naturally to health care professionals, who are conditioned to a more authoritarian model of social change. Medical and paramedical treatment is traditionally authoritarian, for arguably good reasons. The doctor says, 'Take the pills three times a day,' and the patient obeys. Often, the acceptance of the doctor's authority is an important psychological part of the cure, and in spite of Illich and some feminist groups, most people are still happy that this should be so. Curative medicine is a matter, at any given time, for a single patient, whose faith in the treatment can be as significant as the treatment itself.

The case for applying the same model to preventive medicine, however, is much weaker. At one extreme, however much one may feel that society would be the better for drinking less alcohol or none at all, there is nobody left to argue that the USA was the better for Prohibition and Al Capone. Similarly, few doctors would advocate achieving the abolition of car accidents by the abolition of cars.

These may seem absurd and extreme examples, but in a way they are not; for they raise the problem of who is to draw the lines, and where? The confidence shown by official, professional and scientific opinion in every sphere that, whatever the case in the past, it now knows the answers and has only to apply them to solve the problem is not supported by history. The outstanding work of the advertising industry for the Government during World War II in promoting healthier eating in circumstances of severe shortages nevertheless contained the reiterated advice that everyone should 'eat something every day' from a food group which contained all of these items; sugar, butter, margarine, dripping, suet, lard.[5] Walker and Cannon[6] say that such doctrines 'were valuable in their day. But now they are basically outdated.' They do not speculate on what would have been the consequences if such propaganda had been continued through sheer bureaucratic inertia for a further 30 years.

6 The case for freedom of choice

Logically, a case can be made for the abolition of all advertising, even if the practical problems would be immense. What is not acceptable within the context of the society in which we live is the substitution of single-source advertising for multi-source advertising. However worthy the motives, totalitarian propaganda in any medium is a step towards the diminution and ultimate extinction of liberty of thought and expression. As with the press and TV, so with advertising: whatever misgivings we may have about the justice and equity of the present system, it is inconceivable that it will be improved by greater concentration of power into fewer hands, and impossible that any body of Platonic 'guardians' could be trusted indefinitely not to abuse such power. If there is to be progress from the underlying concepts of liberalism inherent in western institutions, it must be towards more, not less, freedom of opinion and expression; more, not less, freedom of choice.

And freedom of choice, as the story of the Garden of Eden is surely meant to demonstrate, includes the freedom to choose wrongly, the freedom to choose evil as well as good. A healthily evolving society is one in which it is possible to explore the risks of alternative choices – even though the consequences are sometimes harmful for some individuals. Consciously to prevent any further experimentation on the part of individuals in the name of safety, hygiene or preventive medicine is to risk halting the future development of mankind dead in its tracks. One generation's blind alley may be the next generation's break-through, and the suppression of heterodox opinion, whether it be that of Galileo, the Abbé Mendel or General Foods, is always likely to make the orthodox look fools in the light of history.

7 Advertising controls – the guarantee of freedom

This is not, of course, an argument for complete individual anarchy. Rules there must be if any society is to exist, let alone survive, and rules of some kind have been accepted by the advertising industry for a very long time.

The present self-regulatory system which governs the greater part of advertising in the UK today should be sufficiently well-known to informed readers not to need much elaboration in this context: at least the advertisements for the Code of Advertising Practice (which covers all printed advertising) can have left few who are interested unaware that advertisements must be 'decent, honest, legal and truthful'. But the point about the Code – and about its TV and radio equivalent, which is intrinsically similar but has statutory backing – is that it is flexible enough to take account of changes of culture and knowledge as they occur – something which legislators and governments find far harder to do – and that it is obeyed for the most part in the spirit as well as the letter: a claim that it would be hard to make for, say, the tax provisions of the Finance Acts.

Significantly, though, the Code assumes the whole competitive nature of the advertising enterprise, and its enforcement body, the independent Advertising Standards Authority, has refused to enforce the Code in the case of political or religious advertising, where no objective assessment of competing claims is even theoretically possible.

Significantly, too, the National Consumer Council finds little to complain of in the Code: its guns are currently trained on those utilities, whether privatised or nationalised, which enjoy monopoly powers. Health educators have been less generous in their assessment. They have pressed for ever tighter restrictions on the advertising of drink, tobacco, and now such foodstuffs as they currently believe to be harmful to the national diet. Yet, having succeeded many years ago in removing cigarette advertising from television, they are confronted with a Frankenstein's monster of their own creation in the form of massive sports sponsorship by the tobacco companies, which costs far less than TV advertising and secures far longer exposure on the screen to far wider and more vulnerable audiences.

And now, although the consumption of tobacco continues to fall gently, the pressure is on to abolish sports sponsorship, as if we could be certain that the ingenuity of tobacco manufacturers in finding ways to sell products which they are legally entitled to make has somehow been exhausted by the popularity of snooker.

8 The alternative to advertising

Advertising people have generally held that there should be freedom to advertise any product or service which can be legally offered for sale. This is, of course, blatant self-interest, not dissimilar to the self-interest of journalists who maintain their right to publish whatever constitutes news, even if it endangers national security.

But it is not, as it is not with journalists, merely self-interest. Far from the myth of 'hidden persuasion', advertising is always open and apparent for what it is: every advertisement is clearly and unmistakeably a biased message on behalf of a product or opinion whose signature it bears, and it is universally recognised for what it is. Not all forms of promotion, not even those employed by pressure groups of unimpeachable virtue, are as morally defensible as the open, undisguised touting of his wares by a producer.

And some form of promotion there will continue to be for any product that is legally produced. As the Soviet government has long discovered, products do not sell themselves, and all the apparatus of communism has not found 'vays of makink you buy' to equal the advertising of branded goods. Soviet advertising, however, emanating from a single government source, knows no code of practice, and commercials are regularly screened in the USSR which would be banned in the UK on the grounds of health and safety. Against the political bias of single-source advertising there can be no appeal.

Moreover, if a market genuinely exists – if the demand is there and the price is right – even goods which are not legitimate will find means of promotion. Prostitution, cannabis and now heroin have flourished without the help of the legitimate persuaders – and without the controls which the advertising industry today accepts with such relatively good grace.

9 The perils of restriction

It may not be universally true, as American neo-conservative analysts such as Glazer have argued, that government policies are liable to foment results exactly opposite to that which their promoters intend. What may be said is that the outcome of legislation – and particularly of restrictive legislation – is sufficiently uncertain to justify an attitude of caution rather than self-righteousness among its promoters.

Labour governments, determined to give tenants a better deal, passed Rent Acts which made rented property almost disappear. The present administration, in its single-minded determination to reduce the volume of public spending, has actually seen it increase year by year. Taxation, annually tinkered with to right supposed wrongs, has spawned a tax avoidance industry which today consumes a great slice of our national income. Much of the recent labelling legislation, here and in the EEC, has failed of its purpose, because it is based on preconceptions about what people *ought* to read, rather than sympathy with what they *want* to read, and the result has often been that they read and understand less than before.

Competitive advertising is one of the few mechanisms for change compatible with a free society, and in consequence it is slow and uncertain. In spite of costly research and planning, most new brands and many new products still fail in the marketplace, and those that succeed may take a decade or more before they are established, only to be swept away by an unpredictable change in taste or fashion. The brilliance of Guinness advertising over half a century could not stem the swing to lager which was initiated, not by scheming brewers or impassioned temperance workers, but by people who had been on foreign holidays and developed a taste for something different.

Mussolini made the trains run on time, and Hitler improved the health of the German people. The price, though, was high. Advertising, like democracy, is tedious and slow: but it is killing fewer people all the time.

Notes and References

1. B.K. Tones, 'The Use and Abuse of Mass Media in Health Promotion' in *Health Education and the Media*, Pergamon, 1981.
2. Examples quoted are from Charles Channon (ed.), *Advertising Works 3*, Holt, Reinhart, 1985.
3. M.J. Waterson MA, *Advertising and Alcohol Abuse*, Advertising Association, 2nd edition, 1983.
4. Michael Binyon, 'Alcohol is Deadliest Internal Threat to Soviet Union', *The Times*, 6th January 1981.
5. *Modern Publicity in War*, The Studio Publications, 1941, pp.39–51.
6. Caroline Walker and Geoffrey Cannon, *The Food Scandal*, Century Publishing, 1984, p.43.

12 Regulating Cakes and Ale: Agricultural Intervention and Health

Catherine Montgomery Blight and Simon Scanlan

1 Introduction

> 'Dost thou think because thou art virtuous,
> there should be no more cakes and ale?'
> (Twelfth Night, Act II, Sc 3)

Thus, Sir Toby Belch put the argument on regulating our diet in a nutshell. The economic justification for the government intervening to change our eating and drinking patterns is that our habits are so bad for us that they lead to illness and consequently a cost on the public purse. As far as alcohol and tobacco are concerned, direct taxes are paid by the consumer, but to control the amount of fat in our diet, an eccentric and devious policy has been adopted, directed towards penalising the producer, rather than the consumer.

This article seeks to challenge the easy assumption that legislation can provide the answer to social problems and to show that in the context of regulating the amount of fat in our diet, the rules which have been adopted have been ill-conceived.

2 Changing eating trends – without legislation

British eating habits have changed, in some cases dramatically, over the last four decades. Put simply, these changes have been brought about by two main influences, socio-economic changes and advertising. The impact of advertising is considered in another chapter. Technological advances in production, distribution and in domestic appliances have all led to a marked increase in the quantity of processed and ready prepared food purchased. Within the family, traditional eating patterns are giving way to more casual, less structured habits. More women working outside the home and at the same time more interest in leisure activities have also given an impetus to the demand for convenience foods. According to the Meat and Livestock Commission, (*Meat Demand Trends* February 1986) household consumption of frozen/chilled convenience meats and meat products and frozen/chilled ready meals has increased steadily and consistently over recent years. Awareness of health considerations in what we eat has led to an increased demand for high fibre products and for organically grown fruit and vegetables. For example, consumption of breakfast cereals has increased from 2.95 ozs per capita per week in 1973 to 3.83 ozs in 1983. These changes have taken place not through enforcement by legislation, but rather through each of us choosing what we want to eat. It is difficult to find an example of a change in eating habits which has actually been the result of direct regulation (apart from food rationing in war-time) – the most obvious one probably is the development of the take-away trade, which followed the imposition of VAT on with-service meals in restaurants.

To sum up, changes in consumer demand, sparked off by changes in life-style, fads or even fashions on the one hand, and changes in the supply-side of food producing and retailing on the other, mean that the kaleidoscope of the market can, and does, constantly react, without the necessity of regulation. In other words, market forces are so powerful that they keep breaking through.

3 Healthier eating?

Despite the popular belief that there is more awareness of the importance of sound nutrition, there has been a marked increase in the consumption of snack foods, fizzy drinks and other fun foods. According to Taylor Neilson Associates, consumption of chocolate biscuits has increased by 33 per cent and of fizzy drinks by 66 per cent over four years. A comment in *Frozen Food – consumer market bulletin 1985* from Ross Foods paints the picture more vividly.

> The other sector which has tended to buck the trend in terms of healthier eating is the traditional Hot Puddings market, now valued at well over £10 million and dominated by products such as Ross Jam and Treacle Roly Polys, Spotted Dick, Apple and Blackberry Dumplings and Bramley Apple Pie. In this respect a yoghurt and an apple five days a week seems, in conscience, to justify at least one week-end treat of Treacle Roly Poly and Custard.

There is though, a more disturbing side to the problem of unhealthy eating than the diseases of sheer gluttony. A recent report by Nicola Bull, on the eating habits of the 15 to 25 year old age group suggests that within that sector of the population, there is some evidence of serious malnutrition. Yet the Government's policy on food and health expenditure is directed towards the wealthier sectors, who over-eat. In fact, there was a trend towards eating less fat even before the publication of the NACNE and COMA reports. In 1973 average total fat consumption per head per week was 11.22 ozs. By 1983, it was 10.69 ozs. In 1973, average butter consumption was 5.24 ozs per head per week. By 1983, it was 3.27 ozs.

Expenditure of public funds on cutting down the amount of fat in our diet is open to challenge. It is probably not needed anyway. However, there are other arguments against what is being done. When we examine how the authorities choose to put the policies into effect, we find a mass of absurd rules and contradictory results.

4 'There ought to be a law...'

First, we must look more closely at how those rules and regulations arise. Underlying the demand for regulation are two assumptions:- that when a problem arises, it is the responsibility of the Government to provide an answer and that the only way to achieve a solution is by legislation. The reaction generally is 'There ought to be a law ...'. What actually happens is that *ad hoc* specific regulations tend to have unexpected results, often perverse or the opposite of what was intended. As long ago as 1971, Professor George Stigler argued that regulation is a process of political exchange between politicians and political parties on the one hand and industrialists and industries on the other. Extending this argument, Professor Israel Kirzner maintains that regulations hinder the market process by actually restraining entrepreneurship and innovation. There is, however, a more sinister and more damaging effect in pandering to the demand for regulation. What can develop is the destruction of the relationship among traders in the market. Negotiations between producers and consumers are impeded. Adjustments through the market process are constrained. Consumer preferences are blurred and producer response is confused.

5 Where do the benefits from regulation go? Not always where you'd expect

It is important at this stage in the discussion to explain in more detail how the regulatory process works. What has actually happened is that a sophisticated and complex phenomenon has emerged. It can be described as a market for regulation superimposed on the market for actual products. It is not just a simple matter of answering the demand 'There ought to be a law ...'. Certainly, the *supply* of the regulation is derived from the legislature and its delegated agencies. It is they who have the power to enact laws, rules and regulations. The *source* of the demand for regulation is any interest which sees a possible advantage in obtaining a particular regulation. In other words, the market for regulation is best understood as part of the competitive process. Regulation therefore occurs because there are well-organised interests which expect to benefit. Trade organisations lobby in Parliament, in the press, through public relations activities. Sometimes, unexpected coalitions arise between, for example, industry and consumer groups, overtly opposed, but covertly acting in concert. From time to time, we see members of interest groups forming associations and disbanding to align with others, as circumstances and motives change. Within this framework, officials and bureaucrats play a subtle role, which is rarely obvious. It manifests itself in the bias which such officials show towards regulatory solutions to problems. A more obvious part is played by the dominant firms in an industry. Several writers argue that specific regulations can be proved to give a competitive advantage to the dominant firm, by raising its rivals' costs. Thus, the much vaunted benefits which accrue to consumers from the recent legislation on food labelling should be taken with more than a pinch of salt. What has happened is that food processing companies have actually accepted rules on labelling which suit them.

However, the most glaring examples of the eccentric results of operating under the market for regulation are to be found in the regulations which have been adopted to try to reduce the amount of fat in our diet, especially in the two products which have been identified as the chief culprits, namely milk and red meat. We now examine these two products in more detail.

6 Milk – don't kill the Russians

Most readers will know that the Common Agricultural Policy (CAP) keeps farmers' output prices high by buying up surpluses and putting them into intervention stores, where they become 'mountains' and 'lakes'. In the case of milk, the EEC buys butter and skim milk powder (SMP) at prices which are fixed annually. Whole milk can be processed into these two constituents. Milk producers can, at any time, sell butter and/or SMP to the intervention authorities at the fixed prices.

Intervention offers a guaranteed 'market' to producers for whatever quantity of milk they choose to produce and process into the appropriate form. So it is not surprising that dairy farmers have taken advantage of new technology and genetic improvement to increase their production. Nobody wants to buy the extra milk at the price levels fixed by the CAP, so it is sold into intervention stores.

Putting butter into public cold stores does at least keep it out of consumers' arteries, but it cannot sit there for ever. Eventually it is sold off cheaply to someone, preferably before it goes rancid. Who is the someone? Very often in the past, he has been a Russian or an Eastern European, whose government has usually been keen to buy cheap EEC food to compensate for the failings of its own agriculture.

Unfortunately the idea of selling bargain butter to the Comrades is becoming unpopular with the electorate of Europe. There are more votes in killing our own people through excess fat consumption than there are in killing Russians that way. So the EEC has developed various ways of handing it out cheaply to ice cream makers, to bakers, to the armed forces and to the general public as a special Christmas present. One of the most recent schemes involved sales of concentrated butter (ghee), which sold mostly to processors because ordinary consumers did not know what to do with it. Between 1973, when we joined the EEC, and 1985 Britain had a special subsidy on all packet butter to keep shop prices down, encouraging consumption.

To summarise the bizarre story of intervention butter so far: the CAP guarantees to buy butter at a high price, so farmers produce more than they otherwise would. At the same time, the governments who run this policy say we should eat less butter.

7 Milk – raising the fat content

There is more. The EEC authorities are attempting to correct the worst absurdities of the CAP for milk, although they are doing it for reasons of economy rather than healthy eating. Intervention is a very costly business for the tax payer. First of all, butter has to be paid for. Secondly, it has to be put into cold storage. Thirdly, while it is in there, interest must be paid on the money used to finance it. Fourthly, it is eventually sold (months, or even years later) at a price much lower than was originally paid for it. In 1986, intervention operations for butter are likely to cost the EEC authorities over £640 million, and for SMP over £275 million. Each tonne of intervention butter this year will take from the European taxpayer about £230, and each tonne of SMP about £100, in storage costs alone. (European Commission internal document, quoted in Agra Europe 31 Jan, 1986.)

Intervention butter is therefore particularly costly. In the last three years, the EEC has attempted to correct the relative attractiveness of butter and SMP intervention in order to save money. It has done this by reducing the intervention price for butter by 12.5 per cent, and raising the prices for SMP by 16 per cent. This change sounds as though it will help to reduce the production of dairy fat. Unfortunately not. As our own Scottish Milk Marketing Board put it, 'Whatever the EEC and diet columnists may say, butterfat remains a valuable constituent in milk products, roughly twice as valuable in fact weight-for-weight as SNF (solids not fat). The price dairy product manufacturers are prepared to pay for extra fat in milk demonstrates this'. [SMMB Milk Bulletin, June 1985] It is true that consumption of low fat milks is increasing, but it remains the SMMB's experience that its most profitable manufacturing outlets for milk are in cream, condensed milk and chocolate crumb!

The SMMB is in no doubt that what its customers want is fat. This message is passed faithfully back to dairy farmers in payments for raw milk. It is only as recently as 1984 that the Milk Boards introduced a system in which farmers receive a premium for production of butter fat.

The outcome of the EEC's reduction in the intervention butter price is that the Milk Boards are encouraged to sell dairy fat to consumers, rather than to sell it to the authorities.

8 Lamb – new regulations will discourage grossly fat carcases, but will impede progress from average to lean

The case of lamb provides an example of a British Government regulation, implemented as a direct response to NACNE/COMA, to reduce the fat content of our food. The new regulation came into effect in January 1986, and although it is too early to be precise about its consequences, it is very likely that it will reduce the production of *very* fat lambs. Unfortunately it will do absolutely nothing to encourage farmers to sell lean lambs rather than *fairly* fat ones; indeed it may well impede the progress already being made in this direction by market forces.

The regulation in question was actually a change in the detail of the measures used to subsidise sheep farmers. The measures work roughly as follows. The price of lambs is determined by the market forces of supply and demand. The Government collects reports on sales of lambs at auction markets throughout Great Britain and calculates the average price for each week. The weekly average market price is then compared with a predetermined 'guide price' for the week. If the market price is below the guide, the Government pays out a subsidy to fill the gap. The subsidy is paid to all farmers who sold lambs in that particular week. In effect, the system guarantees that *on average* farmers' returns (ie market price plus subsidy) will always come up to the guide level.

It is important to a farmer to make sure that he gets the subsidy on the lambs he sells, because it can be very large, and, occasionally, even greater than the market price itself. This occurred in the week of 18 July 1983, when the GB average market price for lambs was 107 p/kg and the subsidy was 120 p/kg. It is more important for the farmer to get the subsidy than it is for him to produce the type of lamb which buyers want. In that same week of 1983, the difference in price between over-weight lambs and light lambs was only 20 p/kg.

Before subsidy can be paid on a lamb, an independent (but Government-funded) grader must certify that it passes the required standard. It is this standard which the Government altered in January 1986 as a response to pressure for a healthy diet. Under the new standard, subsidy will be withheld from a further 2.5 per cent of the fattest lambs, unless farmers alter their production and sell their lambs in a leaner condition. From what has been said above, there is a strong incentive for the farmers to do this, and a step is being taken in what appears to be the right direction.

But we can offer only two cheers for this Government action. Its weakness arises from the fact that under the system, a farmer's priority in marketing must be to meet the requirements of the grader. The requirements of the consumer are secondary. Consider the implications for a sheep farmer's marketing decisions. Broadly, he has two options in marketing his lambs: either he can sell them via a traditional auction market, or he can sell them direct to a wholesaler (or abattoir operator). The great advantage of the second, direct method is that the farmer is paid according to the exact characteristics of the carcase his lambs produce. He has rapid and accurate feedback on how his lambs match consumer requirements, and is therefore more able to respond to a public wishing to reduce its fat intake.

The trouble is that the Government's change in the certification standard works in favour of the first, traditional method of selling. If a lamb fails to meet the standard for subsidy when its carcase is graded in the direct abattoir sale, the farmer can do nothing more about it. In contrast, in the auction sale, lambs are certified live by the grader. If a lamb is judged over-fat, and ineligible for subsidy, the farmer can withdraw it from sale and take it home again to work off some fat, before resubmitting it at a later sale. Now that the Government has made it more difficult to pass the grader, farmers have more incentive to use the auction markets for selling lambs. They will thus not get the direct flow of information which they could from the alternative route. So a supermarket chain wishing to sell very lean lamb will find it that much harder to communicate its requirement to farmers.

To sum up: the Government has acted to stop subsidising the production of very fat lambs, but it continues to treat moderately fat lambs and lean ones exactly alike, and its action may impede the trend towards leanness at this level.

9 Beef – deprive consumers of lean meat or encourage production of fat?
The CAP support mechanisms for beef combine the elements of intervention buying (as with milk) and subsidy payment (as with lamb). Intervention in the market immediately presents the Government with a dilemma: what quality of beef should it buy when it acts to take meat off the market? If it is prepared to buy beef regardless of quality, it is in effect offering a guaranteed market outlet for inferior beef, including very fat beef. Farmers could then choose an easy life producing over-fat carcases to add to an unwanted mountain at a generous, government-fixed price.

For this reason, and others, the Government will not accept over-fat beef into intervention and so avoids encouraging excess fat production. Instead, it buys only good quality, lean beef. Thereby it outrages the nation's butchers by removing a proportion of the most desirable meat from the market, leaving them to sell the poorer, fatter beef which is left to them. Whatever type of beef the Government chooses to accept for intervention, it will be wrong.

Turning to the subsidy payment, the picture is similar to the one outlined for lamb, although the distortions caused are less because the beef subsidy is far smaller in relation to market prices. Again, the Government has altered standards so that it is no longer subsidising very fat beef. But delving a little deeper, we can find further instances where the subsidy system tends to discourage lean carcase production. The basis of beef production in Britain is the steer, ie the castrated male bovine. Steers are likely to be fatter than bulls, so it might be thought that the Government would discourage the practice of castrating male calves. But it does the opposite: bulls cannot qualify for subsidy in the auction market (although they can qualify as carcases in the abattoir). The main reason for this is that graders are not keen to spend time at close quarters with a bull, prodding and feeling it in order to gauge its fatness. (The result is euphemistically known in the trade as 'handling problems'.)

10 Pork – less regulation, less fat

We have given examples from the milk and meat industries to show that agricultural policy is not primarily intended to 'improve' our diet, and that even where that is the intention, the result may not be all that was expected. What happens *without* regulation?

Producers and processors of pork operate without interference from intervention buying and direct subsidies. There are some CAP measures applied to pork but they are trivial in comparison with those for their competitors, beef and lamb. Pig farmers face a relatively free market, where they can survive only by producing what consumers want to buy. So they have been forced to respond to the increasing preference for leanness by producing leaner pigs. Between 1975 and 1984, the depth of the fat layer on the back of the average pig (where pig fat is concentrated) decreased from 17.0 mm to 13.5 mm. The amount of lean meat in a carcase rose from under 48 per cent of total weight, to over 52 per cent. By comparison, the percentage of lean in an average beef carcase rose by a tiny amount from 60.2 in 1976 to 60.3 in 1984. The change in lamb carcases was similarly small, from 55.9 per cent in 1977, to 56.1 in 1984.

The improvement in pig carcases has taken place without any Government regulation to help it. This difference is not the only advantage which the pork industry has over beef and lamb (the pig is a more uniform animal, and pig production is a more controlled process) but it is an important one.

11 Agricultural policy does not encourage healthy eating

In Western Europe, a colossal amount of money is spent on regulating the market for food. Most of it goes into the European Community's Common Agricultural Policy. In 1984/85, £1,780 million was spent on grants and subsidies to UK agriculture, of which £1,424 million was spent on market regulation (ie direct market interference) under the Common Agricultural Policy. The objects of the policy were set out in the Treaty of Rome in 1957 and they have nothing to do with improving diet. Article 39 of the Treaty spells it out more clearly:-

> (a) to increase agricultural productivity by promoting technical progress and by ensuring the rational development of agricultural production and the optimum utilisation of the factors of production, in particular labour;
> (b) thus to ensure a fair standard of living for the agricultural com-

munity, in particular by increasing the individual earnings of persons engaged in agriculture;
(c) to stabilise markets;
(d) to assure the availability of supplies;
(e) to ensure that supplies reach consumers at reasonable prices.

This is current law and it is mandatory. So it is not surprising that surpluses have arisen. What we find even more surprising however, is that no thought has been given to adjusting the terms of the CAP in the proposals presently in train to amend the Treaty. Attention instead is being focussed on such matters as improving the internal market, powers of the European Parliament, environment and many points of procedure. Surely in reassessing the terms of the Treaty any provisions which are themselves exceptions to the Treaty – and that is what the CAP is – ought to be put under the microscope. That, though, is not on the agenda and we are still left with a policy which is aimed at quantity of production rather than quality. Tinkering with regulations within these constraints will only further confuse the markets and create even more obstacles between the consumer and producer.

12 Conclusion

We have argued that current agricultural policy does not encourage healthy eating; we have shown here that the higher the incidence of market interference the less does the resulting product match healthy eating standards; we claim that existing policies on reducing fat are misguided, misinformed and misplaced; and we conclude that to make any significant improvement in our diet what is needed is not more regulation, but less. Sir Toby would surely have agreed.

Notes and References

Catherine Montgomery Blight, 'Demand for regulation on Agricultural Products', paper presented to the British Association for the Advancement of Science, 1985.
Peter Bowbrick, 'The economics of grades', *Oxford Agrarian Studies*, No.XI, 1982.
Nicola Bull, 'Dietary Habits of 15–25 year olds', *Human Nutrition: Applied Nutrition*, Vol. 39A, Supplement 1, 1985.
Martin Grantley-Smith, 'Changes in Carcase Composition during the last decade', *Journal of Animal Production* in press.
Household Food Consumption and Expenditure 1973–1983, HMSO.
Scottish Milk Marketing Board, *Milk Bulletin*, June 1985.

Publications from the Social Affairs Unit

THE WAYWARD CURRICULUM
A CAUSE FOR PARENTS' CONCERN?

'...illustrates how the traditional subjects that formed the basis of the "liberal humane" curriculum in schools for nearly a century after the 1870 Education Act have been perverted for political reasons, by naive teachers in the last 20 years' *Daily Telegraph*

'Dubious lessons damage pupils' *Daily Mail*

'Many teachers are hostile to quality and excellence, have a contempt for grammar, a distaste for mainstream moral and cultural values, are often influenced by Marxism and are obsessed with their own pay and status.

So say 23 teachers, academics and educationists in a book published...by the conservative Social Affairs Unit.

The timetable of many schools is now occupied by "harmful subjects taught by unreliable methods" claim the authors – anti-racism education, peace studies, women's studies are cited as examples.

And many of the traditional subjects "display few of the disciplines traditionally associated with them." ' *Times Educational Supplement*

'Wayward lessons raise academic ire' *The Guardian*

ISBN 0 907631 19 3 £9.95

TAKING THOUGHT FOR THE POOR

WEALTH AND POVERTY: A JEWISH ANALYSIS
Jonathan Sacks

ISBN 0 907631 15 0 £2.00

THE BIBLE, JUSTICE AND THE CULTURE OF POVERTY: EMOTIVE CALLS TO ACTION VERSUS RATIONAL ANALYSIS
Irving Hexham

ISBN 0 907631 16 9 £2.00

THE PHILOSOPHY OF POVERTY: GOOD SAMARITANS OR PROCRUSTEANS
Antony Flew

ISBN 0 907631 17 7 £2.00

THE CHRISTIAN RESPONSE TO POVERTY: WORKING WITH GOD'S ECONOMIC LAWS
James Sadowsky

ISBN 0 907631 18 5 £2.00

'These papers are most enjoyable and readable. They conscientiously adopt unfashionable positions and defend them with clarity and verve. The series is one that deserves to be read.'

Professor Keith Ward, F.D. Maurice Professor of Moral & Social Theology, King's College, London

(of *Wealth and Poverty*)
'I want you all to have read [it] by next Monday...it constitutes (obliquely and not by design) the most devastating criticism of the views which the Christian Churches in the West now regularly proclaim on this matter.'

T.E. Utley *The Daily Telegraph*

'Good advice for the Archbishop's Commission [on inner cities]'

Ronald Butt *The Times*

'An intellectual counter-attack is underway from the Social Affairs Unit.'

Walter Schwarz *The Guardian*

RESEARCH REPORTS

DETERRING POTENTIAL CRIMINALS
Ernest van den Haag

Argues that the prime purpose of punishment should be the long-term deterrence of crime

Research Report 7, ISBN 0 907631 14 2 £2.00

ASIAN HOUSING IN BRITAIN

Jon Davies

'...a broadside attack on academic research into immigrant housing'

New Society

Research Report 6, ISBN 0 907631 13 4 £2.00

REVERSING RACISM: LESSONS FROM AMERICA
Kenneth M. Holland & Geoffrey Parkins

'Britain ...warned today against emulating the American pattern of positive discrimination' *The Times*

Research Report 5, ISBN 0 907631 10 X £2.00

ACTION ON WELFARE: REFORM OF PERSONAL INCOME TAXATION AND SOCIAL SECURITY
Hermione Parker

'...represent(s) an important contribution to the debate on social policy the Government cannot ignore' *The Times*

Research Report 4, ISBN 0 907631 04 5 £2.00

TRACTS BEYOND THE TIMES: A BRIEF GUIDE TO THE COMMUNIST OR REVOLUTIONARY MARXIST PRESS
Charles Ellwell

'I can warmly recommend it...a valuable guide' Bernard Levin *The Times*

Research Report 3, ISBN 0 907631 08 8 £1.50

ARE THE POLICE FAIR? NEW LIGHT ON THE SOCIOLOGICAL EVIDENCE
P.A.J. Waddington

'Sociologists rapped for anti-police bias' *Police Review*
Research Report 2, ISBN 0 907631 07 X £1.00

ARE THE POLICE UNDER CONTROL?
David Regan

'a good case' *Daily Telegraph*
Research Report 1, ISBN 0 907631 06 1 £1.00

COLLECTIONS

TRESPASSING? BUSINESSMEN'S VIEWS ON THE EDUCATION SYSTEM
Michael Brophy et al.

'...much of what the industrialists say would be readily embraced by people in the LEAs and activists in the teaching profession' *Education*

ISBN 0 907631 11 8 £2.95

HOME TRUTHS
Barbara Robson et al.

'illustrate(s) the need for members to be aware of the chasm that too often yawns between even progressive housing policies and how they work out in practice' *Local Government Chronicle*

ISBN 0 907631 05 3 £2.95

EDUCATED FOR EMPLOYMENT?
Digby Anderson et al.

'...the (SAU) has turned its attention to the need for a more precisely governed relationship between educator and employer' *Times Higher Education Supplement*

ISBN 0 907631 03 7 £2.65

THE PIED PIPERS OF EDUCATION
Antony Flew et al.

'The SAU has chosen a provocative role in an attempt to improve real debate about the ground rules for education and welfare' *Times Educational Supplement*

ISBN 0 907631 02 9 £2.65

CRIMINAL WELFARE ON TRIAL
Colin Brewer et al.

'Its new and astringent mix of pragmatism and genuine social concern…is bound to attract a positive response' *Church Times*

ISBN 0 907631 01 1 £2.65

BREAKING THE SPELL OF THE WELFARE STATE
Digby Anderson, June Lait & David Marsland

'almost as critical of the present government's strategies as the policies of previous Labour administrations' *The Guardian*

ISBN 0 907631 00 2 £2.65

DETECTING BAD SCHOOLS: A GUIDE FOR NORMAL PARENTS
Digby Anderson

'combines sense with humour…never dull…if it alerts parents to their rights…and reminds teachers of their responsibilities to parents, it can do a lot of good' *Universe*

ISBN 0 907631 04 5 £1.00

EXTRA DRY: COLUMNS IN THE TIMES
Digby Anderson

'imperative writing on political and social subjects' *The Spectator*

ISBN 0 907631 12 6 £2.95

Commissioned by the SAU and published by SPCK

THE KINDNESS THAT KILLS: THE CHURCHES' SIMPLISTIC RESPONSE TO COMPLEX SOCIAL ISSUES

Digby Anderson (ed.)

'rightly censures the clerical fashion which has so superficially equated Christianity with the clichés of socialism'

Ronald Butt, *The Times*

'an excellent point of reference...sets out succinctly the feebleness, predictability, ignorance and uncharitableness of so many church productions' Charles Moore, *The Spectator*

'suggests the true point that the Bible ends in the vision of the City of God, not in the editorial offices of *The Guardian*'

David Edwards, *Church Times*

ISBN 0 281 04096 6 £3.95

Just Published

FAMILY PORTRAITS

Mary Kenny on Feminists and the Family
Robert Chester on the popularity of the 'normal' family
Patricia Morgan on feminists' attempts to sack fathers
Hermione Parker on government subversion of the family
Duncan Mitchell on artificial reproduction and the future of the family and *David Marsland* on young people and the state, *Valerie Riches* on permissiveness, *Andrew Brown* on the family in 'permissive' Sweden and *Digby Anderson* and *Graham Dawson* on the popular but unrepresented 'normal' family.

ISBN 0 907631 20 7 £4.95

The Social Affairs Unit

The Unit is a research and educational trust committed to the promotion of lively and wide-ranging debate on social affairs and to the sociological analysis of key controversies in contemporary culture. Its recent programme has included studies of social service reform, the relation of higher education and business and enterprise, secondary school standards, police accountability and effectiveness, housing, ethnic minorities, criminal deterrence and rehabilitation, the media and the churches and social issues. All Unit publications represent the views of their individual authors, not those of the Unit. Many of them contribute to debates on rapidly changing social issues; they inevitably reflect the circumstances at the time of writing. The Unit's work is assisted by an advisory council which includes:

Unit publications and further information may be obtained from The Social Affairs Unit, Two Lord North Street, Westminster, London SW1P 3LB Telephone: 01-799 3745